Mel Stangeland holds a Ph.D. in clinical neuropsychology and is now retired after a 48-year career working as a psychologist in the fields of mental health and forensic psychology. He resides in British Columbia, Canada. He has always enjoyed learning about new things, travel and the arts. This is his first published work.

This is dedicated to my wife, Terry, whose creative thinking inspired many of the concepts in this book.

Mel Stangeland

THE MECHANIC'S GUIDE TO THE HUMAN PSYCHE

AUSTIN MACAULEY PUBLISHERS®

LONDON * CAMBRIDGE * NEW YORK * SHARJAH

Ordering Information
Quantity sales: Special discounts are available on quantity purchases by corporations, associations, and others. For details, contact the publisher at the address below.

Publisher's Cataloging-in-Publication data
Stangeland, Mel
The Mechanic's Guide to the Human Psyche

ISBN 9798889101048 (Paperback)
ISBN 9798889101055 (ePub e-book)

Library of Congress Control Number: 2024921643

www.austinmacauley.com/us

First Published 2024
Austin Macauley Publishers LLC
40 Wall Street, 33rd Floor, Suite 3302
New York, NY 10005
USA

mail-usa@austinmacauley.com
+1 (646) 5125767

As we progress through life, we encounter many ideas that shape our perspective on life, and we generally cannot remember where those ideas came from. There have, however, been a couple of influences that have stood out for me. The first is the late Dr. Park Davidson, whose undergraduate lectures on personality theory were a starting point in my journey towards a more comprehensive understanding of human behavior. The second is Jane Roberts' book *The Nature of Personal Reality*. The third is the life stories of the many clients that I saw over the years who were willing to openly share their experiences. And, most importantly, the influence of my life partner who has always been able to come up with new perspectives.

Table of Contents

A little while and I will be gone from among you, whither I cannot tell. From nowhere we came, into nowhere we go. What is life? It is a flash of a firefly in the night. It is a breath of a buffalo in the winter time. It is as the little shadow that runs across the grass and loses itself in the sunset.

Dying words of Chief Crowfoot, overlooking the Bow River, 25 April 1890.

Chapter 1
Introduction

I prepared the bulk of this manuscript around 1980. At that time, I was employed as a clinical psychologist in a mental health center in a small rural community. Probably because of a lack of confidence and unfamiliarity with the world of book publishing, I never did anything further with it. It sat on a back shelf while I went on to work another six years in mental health before completing a Ph.D. in clinical neuropsychology. While doing so, I became employed in the field of forensic psychology and maintained a private practice that included forensic assessments, head injury evaluations, psychotherapy, neurofeedback training, and custody and access evaluations. All of this came to an end when I recently retired. Now I have the time to reconsider what I wrote so many years ago.

Writing this book was, and is, an attempt to distill the essence of personal learning in the fields of psychology, philosophy, and theology. I am not referring simply to academic learning, but to learning that grows out of personal experience. Wisdom arising from experience is, of course, always guided by a framework of theory but theory means little if it cannot be connected to experience. My experience has come through a variety of sources that have included some unusual opportunities.

One important source of experience has been my work in the field of psychology. This has allowed me the opportunity to share the personal worlds of thousands of individuals. I have considered it a privilege to be a witness to the human struggle for dignity, meaning, and happiness. In particular, there have been some individuals whose intensity, persistence, and resilience have been an inspiration. Being exposed to the inner experiences of other people of various cultural and ethnic backgrounds has allowed opportunities to see the universal experiences of thought and emotion. Speaking with others in such a personal way has also served as a mirror for me, permitting me to see parts of myself as a manifestation of the universal human experience.

My learning has also come through exposure to the ideas of many people, both through books and through personal communication. I have tended toward an independent attitude that leaves me reluctant to accept any idea as true unless I have evaluated it against my own experience. Thus, the ideas that are presented here are those to which I feel a deep commitment. They are ones that I have found to be personally valuable and worthy of consideration for searchers in the human journey.

Of all the individuals from whom I have learned, none has been more important than my wife, Terry. Many of the ideas that follow are the direct result of her creative thinking and insight. She continually demonstrates the levels of creativity and insight that are possible if one is willing to trust their intuition.

It is not my intention to present a comprehensive theory of human behavior or in any way to expand the limits of knowledge in the fields of psychology, sociology, philosophy, or theology. Viewing this work as a theory would intellectualize and depersonalize it and limit its value as a tool for growth. Instead, it is my hope that you might begin to see that you are the theory and that, in order to understand those around you, you must begin to understand yourself. I hope that you will begin to see that the pathway to understanding all things lies within your thoughts, feelings, and experiences.

This lesson was best exemplified for me when, in 1967, I first encountered a group of people who were involved in Zen meditation. I was young and not in a very good mental state at the time. I was curious but afraid. I wanted to know what to expect if I were to try meditation. I kept asking, "What is supposed to happen when you meditate?" The only answer I ever received was, "Meditate and find out." It was frustrating because I wanted an explanation and a tour guide, but I never received one. A few months later, I was in a state of anxiety and depression. I felt alone and lost. I decided to follow the advice I had been given, so I bought a short book called *Yoga Meditation* by Richard Hittleman. It gave some simple exercises to do as a starting point, such as staring at a candle or an object with the focus on the breath or breathing in deeply and repeating the word Om on the out-breath.

What transpired from there was life-changing for me. I experienced a radical change in my emotional state. I felt calmer and more able to focus on the moment instead of on my fears. I strongly recommend meditation but I would emphasize that no one's experience is ever exactly the same as anyone else's. So, my advice would be to 'meditate and find out'.

One of the teachings of the Buddhist philosophy that is worth trying to understand is that human suffering and unhappiness arise out of attachment. By attachment, I mean the belief that something is very important or necessary in our lives. This can be an attachment to material possessions, but it can also be an attachment to ideas and circumstances, all of those things that we hold to be part of our working reality. The attachments may be so much a part of our psyche that we may not even recognize them. We want to hold on to what we have, but the material world is constantly changing. We are immersed in a never-ending river of change. Nothing remains constant, including us. When we cling to our possessions, experiences, and perceptions, we open ourselves to disappointment, frustration, and pain by attempting to stem the tide of change. When we seek our happiness through things that are external to ourselves, we place ourselves at the mercy of this ever-changing flow. We delight at newfound prosperity, status, possessions, and relationships but despair at their loss.

Our lives become a cycle of alternating hope and despair. Most of us approach our lives with a kind of stock market mentality. When the market is up, we are happy, but when the market is down, we are stressed, anxious, or depressed. We are at the mercy of our circumstances.

Many of us are living in an age of security wherein we hope that we will be able to end the cycle of change by accumulating sufficient material goods and comforts to prevent despair. This plan is, however, vulnerable to uncontrollable circumstances, such as inflation, recession, the energy crisis, pollution, pandemics, overpopulation, and the winds of war. There is no security when we seek our happiness in things external to ourselves.

By seeking to understand our thoughts, feelings, needs, beliefs, and values it becomes possible to see life in a different way. It allows us to make what is known as a second-order change. This kind of change can be illustrated by imaging yourself as a queen on a chess board. All around you, you see friends and enemies moving about, creating situations that threaten you or create freedom for you. It all seems quite confusing. There is no basis by which to decide how to move other than the immediate consequences. A second-order change in this situation would allow you to see yourself as participating in a game that has rules and a purpose. You would see that you are playing a role in this game and that each other piece also has a role to play. You would see that the most valuable aspect of the game is the experience that is gained with each new game.

It is when we are able to make this kind of second-order change that we can begin to experience real freedom. When we are able to see that we are the perceivers and, as such, we have the freedom to give our own meaning to our reality, we will have taken an important step toward liberation.

The discussions in the following chapters are intended to help you look at the way in which you construct reality so as to give you some tools for change. You might think of it as an owner's manual that allows you to explore aspects of your mind and make changes, just like your car manual tells you how to change a tire. Each of the topics discussed opens the avenue to seeing that it is possible to change your perception of the events of your life so that they can be used to promote your personal growth. They also encourage a higher level of awareness of the internal constructs that you use to guide your experience and make it possible to create a new life based on your unique needs and thoughts. The only right answers are the ones that are meaningful to you. You are the creator.

I have found it important in my personal search to accept that birth and death are gates rather than boundaries. I believe that each of us is a being whose existence is continuous. This is clearly reflected in many of the statements I make. So also is my belief that our universe is the creation of a Supreme Being. I recognize that this may be unpalatable to readers who have closed their minds to such possibilities. However, these assumptions are too fundamental to the ideas presented to avoid. I do not like dogmatism and recoil from any suggestions that a particular set of beliefs must be accepted.

I do not pretend to have any ultimate answers about spirituality or our relationship with God. I am not affiliated with any organized religion. But I believe that it is important to be open to spiritual experiences and to find an inner connection to the spiritual realm. If we can be open-minded, our spiritual understanding will become a part of our personal growth.

I can share a story that had a big impact on me when I think about spirituality. When we lived in that small rural community, we would take our two children every Christmas and travel to the city where our parents lived. After one particular Christmas, we set out to return home on the afternoon of New Year's Eve. We had a small car and had a box attached to the roof to carry suitcases and other things. It was a bitterly cold day with temperatures that would reach about -30 F. With the wind chill, it was much colder. As we headed toward the Rocky Mountains, the wind was blowing so strong against us that I could only do 30 mph. We had to travel through a long stretch of wilderness where no one lived. When we reached the next town, I was reluctant to buy gas there because the price was always so high. I knew there was a discount gas station a little further on, but when we got there, it was closed. I thought of the next place further down the road, but it was also closed. I thought of another place up ahead, but it was closed also. We were still about 30 miles from the next town when the engine started to miss. I sensed disaster.

There was almost no traffic on the road. We would not be able to stay in the car because we would freeze without heat. I said to my wife, "I think we might run out of gas."

She asked, "How much further can we go?" and I said, "I think this is about it." The snow was piled high on each side of the road, but she spotted a street light on the other side of the bank and said, "This must be a farm. Pull in here." I drove through the break in the snow bank and believe it or not, it was a small country gas station. The car stalled about 30 feet from the pumps. The gas station was closed, but through the window, I could see that there were some people gathered in the back of the building for a New Year's Eve party. I knocked on the door and someone came and turned on the pumps for us. I pushed the car to the pump and we were saved. What are the chances of ending up 30 feet from a gas pump in a very isolated area after having traveled over 200 miles? Was this just incredibly good luck? It has always felt like there was something else at play. I think most people have had experiences such as this, where intuition or some unusual circumstance has altered their life trajectory.

Life is an illusion. All that we see as being tangible or real is merely a highly organized pattern of energy. At the level of the atoms and molecules that make up our physical world, there is no physical matter, only patterns of energy. And yet we see what they make as being solid. Regardless, it is a beautiful world. The realization of its illusionary nature opens the door to the existence of many other realities that have their own validity. Realizing that life is an illusion does not mean that you should not take it seriously. Life is a special opportunity for learning and experience. Seeing it as an illusion merely emphasizes the importance of making the most of it.

Each of our minds is like an eye looking out upon reality. What we see depends upon the quality of our sight. When our self-awareness is limited, our vision is poor. We see shadowy forms that frighten us. We flee from them toward glittering lights which seem to offer safety. We seem to be at the mercy of things that we do not understand. We experience fear and uncertainty.

As our self-awareness grows, we can begin to see more clearly. When we see that we are creating the interpretations that give our perceptions meaning, we become free to alter those perceptions. Freed of judgments and evaluation, our perceptions begin to have a softness that was previously unknown. Being free of the need to interpret our perceptions leaves us surrounded by a soft, warm, loving environment.

Life is joy. All the experiences of our life are founded on love and joy. It is through the structuring of reality by our thinking that this joy is lost. From the time of our birth, we are subjected to a hypnotic trance within which we are taught to think about ourselves and our reality. This mental structure then substitutes for the joy of pure being. I hope that this book can in some way help you to find joy in your life.

Chapter 2
The Inner Self

The heathen tell us that 'know thyself' was an oracle that came down from heaven. Sure I am it is this oracle that will lead us to the God of heaven.

W. Secker, 1660

The material that will be presented to you in this book has been designed to assist you in developing a greater awareness of yourself and your life events. It is based on the assumption that life is your own personal creative experience. It is your opportunity to develop your personality in any way you choose. The foundation of life is growth.

Before we begin, I would like to share some thoughts about the existence of a higher power. At one point, I was taking a chemistry course as part of an application to medical school. The professor discussed the concept of entropy. Essentially, entropy is a measure of the disorder or randomness of a system. It is presumed that systems will evolve to a state of homogeneity that maximizes entropy. That is, systems will deteriorate to a state of disorganization over time. The professor compared a number of blocks scattered randomly to a column of blocks. It has taken some form of energy to create the column and, therefore, it possesses a type of potential energy. The concept of entropy suggests that, in the absence of external intervention, physical systems should be prone to decline and decay. Think of what happens to abandoned buildings or life-less planets.

The force that opposes such decline is life. Where there is life, there is growth, order, and organization. Trees and plants produce structure, flowers, and reproductive material. Animals form bodies, build nests, and create offspring. They also create structures (e.g., coral reefs, termite nests). Humans build buildings and create housing, vehicles, electronics, furniture, and so on. Clearly, the force that works in opposition to the concept of entropy is life. Where there is life, there is organization. But what is life? Science has been unable to create life from non-living materials. We can describe the differences between living and non-living things but what creates life is a mystery. Any attempts to artificially create life have been unsuccessful.

In my mind, the existence of life is a strong argument to suggest that there is a force beyond the physical world, a force that we might think of as being God. I feel that attempts to describe God through religious dogma generally fall upon the error of characterizing God in human terms, such as an old man with a beard. Personally, I do not think that the human mind is capable of understanding what God really is, but accepting that such a force is present opens up the prospect of understanding some of the unusual experiences that are not easily accounted for in any other way.

Coming back to the issue of growth, it is a process that must take place, no matter how slowly, or death will occur. Our physical growth is far less important than our spiritual and psychological growth. In our lives here, we are presented with a very special opportunity to experience and learn from our experiences. We are like seeds that have been planted in fertile soil. It might seem that some are in more fertile soil than others, but if experience is what is important, the usual standards of 'the good life' do not apply. Everything that we need to grow is all around us. All we have to do is push out a few roots and accept that which is available to us.

The material in this book is also based on the idea that life is a multifaceted experience. Our day-to-day conscious experience of life is only one aspect of our consciousness. Our consciousness extends beyond that narrow band of logical, sequential experience into other areas that our logical minds have difficulty comprehending. Our consciousness extends into areas where time does not exist, where the future exists before it happens, where the past is changeable, where physical laws do not apply, and where our playful imaginations are free to create any possibility. These aspects of consciousness are available to us through our experiences of dreaming, fantasy, imagination, and psychic experiences. These aspects also make important contributions to our growth and development.

However, before these other areas can be utilized effectively, it is important to first realize that your conscious experience is fully under your conscious/unconscious control. This is not to say that you should understand this intellectually. Rather, it is to suggest that you should know this in the sense of feeling and experiencing the truth of it. The life that you are experiencing now is an experience that you have created through the interplay of the many different aspects of your consciousness.

A natural response to this statement would be to incredulously ask, "If that is true then why am I not rich, happy, and healthy? Why do misfortunes keep happening to me?" If you accept that spiritual and psychological growth are the most important products of your life experience, the answer becomes clear. Utopia would be stagnation. Perfection is static and unchanging. Growth requires a flowing, changing environment that brings new challenges and new perceptions. This need not be painful. The pain comes when we stubbornly refuse to make changes and when we refuse to grow.

Central to the discussion that follows is the idea that your personality is the expression of an entity whose existence goes beyond the boundary of death. It is the expression of an entity that is striving for increasing levels of understanding and love. This entity occupies the body which you see as yourself and is the thinking, feeling being whom you identify as yourself. It also has expression in other realities and dimensions of reality. This entity will be referred to as your true self or your inner self.

Your present personality is a product of the interaction of this entity and the psychological and physical environment in which it is immersed. You, as an entity, have entered the life cycle for your own unique and personal reasons. You have goals that you hope to accomplish that involve the development of different aspects of yourself. The environment in which you find yourself provides opportunities for growth in those aspects. The entities who have served as your parents and family members are suited to facilitating certain kinds of growth within you. You may not be consciously aware of your goals, but they may be sensed intuitively and your natural interests may provide clues that can help you discover them. Life provides a special opportunity for you to have experiences that will contribute to your development.

Experiences produce new learning and new understanding which, in turn, produce new experiences that can stimulate further learning. It is the quality of this interactive sequence of experience and learning that constitutes personal growth. When high growth is taking place, experiences are producing much new learning that produces quality experiences. If you are interested in definitions, you can think of learning as being a first-order construct, whereas growth is a second-order concept, which is defined by the quality of the interaction between learning and experience.

When you begin to understand that reality is what you make it, you will have taken an important step toward growth. If you realize that you are constantly creating your reality, you will be able to greatly enhance the growth that arises out of your experiences and learning. We all accept the idea that experience produces learning. Throughout our years we have heard the expression, 'live and learn'. But to what extent do we see the reverse process, that learning produces new experiences? We treat our learning in an academic way. Information is filed away without much thought about the doors it might open or the ways in which it might be used to create new experiences. The recognition that you are creating experiences is vital for growth to take place.

What will be presented now is a model that may help you gain an understanding of your present personality. It forms the basis for the material that follows so you may wish to refer back to it at various times. As you will see, the underlying concept is really very simple. It is one that can be easily understood at an intellectual level. However, understanding it intellectually will be of very little value to you unless that understanding is accompanied by an awareness of how this applies to your own life. This awareness can come through the thoughts that are generated by the exercises presented.

The core of each of our personalities is the true self or inner self, which is the entity that was referred to earlier. It transcends our existence in the material world and extends beyond the boundaries of birth and death. It is the psychic energy that breathes life into our physical bodies during life and that will retain the knowledge accumulated in life after death occurs. It is rather like a traveler who agrees to visit a foreign land and, in doing so, to abide by certain rules and restrictions that are created by the nature of life in that land. Upon its entry into life, this true self retains no conscious knowledge of its existence prior to life, nor of any of its previous learning (although there are instances where young children remember past lives before losing those memories as they age). Such knowledge is available at another level of consciousness, which may be reached in dreams, trance states, hypnotic regression, and psychic experiences.

However, at this point, becoming aware of this knowledge is not important. You have entered life in a state of not knowing for a reason. This state allows you the freedom to explore your life experiences with a freshness that would not be otherwise possible to achieve. It allows you to focus your attention fully and completely on the life you are living now. It allows you to creatively seek out new possibilities to stimulate growth in areas that have not previously been explored.

But in life, we must take on an identity. Imagine for a moment that you find yourself floating in space (without the obvious problems of survival). You have no name, no possessions, nobody to relate to, no history, no occupation or profession. You are simply consciousness with nothing but your physical form. How would you react? I think most people would react with a sense of panic because they would not know who they are. In other words, they would have no ego or sense of definition of self.

In the early stages of life, we are in a similar state, and events are experienced in a pure form. Perceptions are not subject to judgments and evaluations. Imagine what the world of an infant is like. Without awareness of progressive changes taking place within itself and in the world around it, time would not exist for the infant. There would be no concept of the future or the past, but only a total focus on the experience of the here and now. There are no thoughts or beliefs to structure experience so that all things are possible. There are no limits and no categories by which events can be defined. There is no fear or anxiety about what the future might bring. There is no guilt or anger about events of the past. There is only innocent observation of what is. There is an open-mindedness that is willing to accept whatever is perceived as being the nature of the world into which it is entering. The experience of infancy is personally best captured by the memory of our daughter as a baby spending hours examining a single hair, never seeming to tire of it.

However, with increasing experience and the development of language, judgments, and evaluations begin to be attached to events. One of the first evaluations the child makes is that some experiences are pleasurable whereas others are unpleasant or painful. This is the beginning of the concept of good and bad. This concept is then used to evaluate other experiences in the child's life. He (or insert she) begins to generalize and judge many things as good or bad, including himself. He gradually becomes less open and less free in his experience because of the judgments he now makes. He has a tremendous urge to understand the world around him. However, the teaching he receives also serves to close off many other ways of understanding his environment. The growth of his conceptual world leads him further and further from the total openness that he once possessed.

Children often seem to possess an amazing intuitive understanding of others. However, somewhere along the way they frequently seem to lose this, perhaps because they are taught to distrust their inner knowledge. Children have difficulty resisting the lessons that are taught to them by their parents, teachers, and other adults. They gradually accept the thoughts and ideas of their mentors while still retaining some fragments of uniqueness. Through this process, limitations begin to be imposed on the inner self as to what it is able to experience. The inner self's contact with people, things, and events is filtered through a screen of judgments based on concepts such as good/bad and possible/impossible.

This is not intended as a criticism of parenthood, but merely as a description of what is. As a parent, I know the joy of helping my children discover the world around them. I also know that I have passed on to them many of the limitations of my own perceptions. If we can begin to see where we have accepted limitations in our experience, we can open up new possibilities for growth.

Through the child's learning, he/she begins to develop ideas that remain constant from one situation to the next. This provides some stability to his thoughts and gives him some ability to predict his environment. These ideas will be referred to as beliefs, but could, just as easily, be called mental sets or habitual patterns of thinking. These beliefs serve as the basic building blocks in the construction of the individual's reality. Whereas these beliefs initially grow out of the child's learning and experience, they later serve the function of directing, limiting, and creating the individual's experience. They dictate what is desirable and undesirable, what is possible and impossible, what is necessary and unnecessary, what we should seek and avoid, and what we can expect to happen in our lives.

When beliefs become fixed and unchanging, the individual begins to be limited in the ways in which he can perceive his experiences. There is little new learning that grows out of his experiences so future experiences tend to be repetitive. It becomes necessary for the individual to fit his experiences into his beliefs rather than allowing his beliefs to be shaped by his experiences. Growth does not take place because there is no interaction between experience and learning. Since little new learning is taking place, there is no material with which to create new experiences. The lack of new experiences prevents learning. Let us consider some examples of this process.

Almost everyone has encountered an angry, rebellious person whose experiences have led him (or her) to believe that no one will listen to him or that no one cares about him. When this belief is firmly established, he treats others in a way that anticipates an uncaring response from them. He expects that he will not be listened to. He becomes rude and threatening to everyone regardless of his knowledge of them. His belligerence toward others stimulates a belligerent response. There is no growth taking place. Instead, there is only a repetitive cycle in which no new learning takes place and no new experiences are created. His experience is being shaped by his beliefs and serves to confirm those beliefs.

Another example is of a person who believes that he is not as worthy as others. He believes that his own thoughts, feelings, and needs are not as important as those of others. Because of this belief, he always places the needs of others ahead of his own. He finds that his needs are seldom met, but his belief prevents him from asking for consideration from those who could meet them. The inattention of others confirms his belief in his unworthiness. He believes that if others thought of his needs as important, they would recognize and meet them without any communication on his part. The experiences created by his failure to value his own needs confirm his belief in his unworthiness. His experiences are being shaped by his beliefs, but are not changing the belief. There is, again, no effective interaction between belief and experience. No growth is taking place.

Another way in which beliefs affect experience is by blocking out opportunities for certain types of experience. Without consciously realizing it, we may have a number of things that we tell ourselves must not happen in our lives.

I must not fail

I must not become angry.

I must not experience pain.

I must not die.

I must not be humiliated.

I must not anger others.

I must not be weak.

I must not be helpless.

I must not displease a certain person.

I must not experience uncertainty.

These are only a few examples of the types of beliefs that close off areas of experience. A very obvious illustration that touches everyone to one degree or another is cultural expectations of sex role behavior. Important areas of experience can be closed off through beliefs as to what is and what is not appropriate sex role behavior. A man who believes that he should not participate in childcare activities denies himself opportunities to express his capacity for nurturance. A woman who believes that her husband should make most of the decisions denies herself the experience of self-sufficiency and independence.

Fears can be thought of as beliefs that impose limits on experience. The emotion of fear is an expression of the belief that certain things must not happen. Whenever you experience fear, you can be aware that you are closing off certain possibilities. You are telling yourself that you will be unable to cope with the events that you are anticipating.

Beliefs also limit the learning that comes through experience when they lead to narrow-mindedness. This occurs whenever anyone is so convinced that his beliefs are correct that he allows no room for change in his ideas. Rigid and inflexible beliefs require that their holder deny or refuse to acknowledge anything that conflicts with these beliefs. A good example of this is the stereotyped beliefs that racial bigots hold about members of another race. Their selective perception allows them to see only those things that confirm their beliefs. In psychology, there is the concept of confirmation bias. This means that we tend to attend to information that confirms what we already hold to be true and ignore information that suggests the opposite.

All of us have certain cherished beliefs that we are very reluctant to change. They may be beliefs about us, about our health, about our past or future, about our life circumstances, about our abilities, and so on. They may be about someone close to us or about groups or society. They may be about our physical environment. Many of our most cherished beliefs are so insidiously interwoven with and fundamental to our thoughts that it becomes very difficult to identify them.

There is no guaranteed safeguard against narrow-mindedness. At one time it was thought that education would create openness, but many highly educated people are very narrow-minded. We look upon science with awe as its technological advances have led us into new areas of experience. However, science has produced its own form of dogmatism in which only the most concrete and tangible phenomena are studied and all else is denied. The only safeguard against narrow-mindedness is to be willing to openly listen to anything that conflicts with your beliefs and to be willing to change the beliefs you now hold.

Needs serve the purpose of focusing the experience of the inner self on selected areas. They provide the vehicle whereby the Self selects from the infinite range of potential experiences, those events that will allow for the development of certain aspects of the self. Thus, through the development of values, beliefs, and needs, a structure is created that allows the inner self to experience a unique, personal conception of reality. This structure becomes the interface through which the inner self experiences reality. It is this structure that creates meaning for the inner self and its interaction with the world in which it finds itself. It is the screen through which the infinite range of potential experiences is filtered in order to determine the actual events of the individual's life. This is commonly known as the ego.

The accompanying diagram provides a visual representation of the mental structure that stands between the inner self and the infinite pool of potential experiences. The mental structure that surrounds the inner self is one's personal reality. The meaning that we apply to our perceptions is provided by that mental structure. Without it, we would experience reality as the newborn infant would experience it. We would experience it as pure perception with no meaning and with infinite possibilities. This mental structure of needs, beliefs, and values is the material by which we create reality.

Lying beyond the mental structure is the infinite pool of potential experiences. Each ring of the mental structure could be thought of as being like walls that contain a variety of gates. In order for a potential experience to pass through a gate, it must meet certain conditions of the gate. It must fall into certain need categories; it must conform to accepted beliefs; and it must agree with prevailing values. If this potential experience is able to meet these tests, then it will be allowed to pass through the gates and be experienced as an event by the inner self.

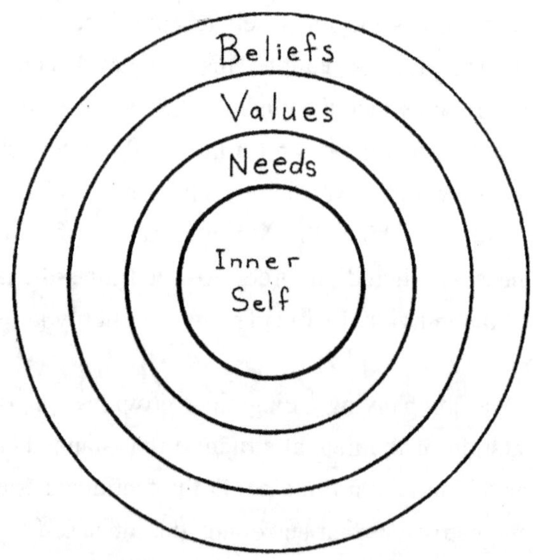

The construction of the mental structure and the experience that is thereby created is the creative expression of the inner self. The construction is never finished. As growth takes place, changes are made in the mental structure. New needs are explored. New beliefs open up event potentials previously unknown. Our creation of reality is an ongoing process. A flexible mental structure facilitates the creative process and enriches the growth of the inner self.

This is not to suggest that all experiences are created through the mental structure. All of us are immersed in a swirling river of forces and influences, some of which are in our control and some of which are outside of our control. At any time, experiences can be forced upon an individual through natural disasters, war, economic changes, sociopolitical events, occurrences in our social group, and so on. Even within such a climate, however, the individual continues to filter these influences and create their personal experiential world.

Much of what follows is aimed at assisting you to become more aware of your own mental structure and to make that mental structure as flexible as possible. When this is accomplished, you will begin to find growth through new learning a daily experience. When you feel highly aware of and capable of changing your mental structure, you can begin to use an expanded awareness of yourself that reaches into other dimensions of experience.

Bear in mind that this book is not intended merely to entertain you. It is aimed at the serious-minded individual who wishes to gain a greater understanding of himself or herself. To get the most out of it, the time you spend completing the exercises will be very important. There is only one person who can possess a complete knowledge of you and that is you yourself. The exercises are a tool that you may use to help you discover your own answers. Their importance lies only in the extent to which they can stimulate and guide your thinking about yourself. Inner knowledge is only gained through self-evaluation, not through any theory or philosophy. Among the early Greeks, a popular counsel was 'know thyself'. What is to follow is a guide for accomplishing that task.

Chapter 3
Self-Acceptance

Over time, I have come to see that the first step in changing ourselves is the development of a measure of self-acceptance and a feeling of self-worth. Invariably, the people I have seen with serious emotional and psychological problems have aspects of themselves—thoughts, feelings, needs—that they are ashamed of and unable to accept. Few of these people could think of themselves in a positive way. Most people have aspects of their thoughts and feelings that they feel they need to cover up or hide. It is obvious that we do not look after, repair, or maintain the objects which we do not value. If we stop valuing something, we allow it to fall into disrepair. The same is true for ourselves. If we do not value our being, we will not care to bring our lives into a state of wellness.

There is a strong tendency to feel that our worth depends upon the value ascribed to us by others. Consequently, rather than acknowledging and acting upon our true thoughts, feelings, and needs, we may put these aside out of the fear that others may disapprove. There is a strong tendency to adopt the trends, values, beliefs, and behaviors that are generally seen as desirable or acceptable.

When our actions are focused on gaining acceptance and adhering to what is socially desirable, it makes personal growth more difficult. It prevents the honest exploration of important areas of experience and closes off growth in those areas. As one is able to accept the thoughts, feelings, and needs that fall outside the range of social approval as being a part of the self, they can be reintegrated and become a valid area for growth.

Most people give up the power to judge themselves early in childhood when they perceive the message that their feelings are less important than the judgment of adults or their peers. In childhood, they forsake many of their natural feelings and judgments about their experience and adopt the ideas and feelings of their parents, teachers, important adults, or their peer group. Social media has only increased this tendency as people look to 'influencers' to tell them what is important.

Let us consider some examples of how this might occur. First, consider Tim, a well-behaved boy whose parents are proud of his trouble-free behavior. They frequently praise him for this and tell others about how easy he is to raise. The external expectation that Tim experiences is contained in his parent's statement, "Our Tim is always so well behaved. He never gets angry about anything." When his natural feeling is anger, it does not match the expectations of his parents. There needs to be a change of perception on the part of Tim or his parents. If Tim's parents are not sensitive to his needs or are persistent in their expectations, Tim may try to bring his feelings into line with the external expectations by modifying his feelings.

When children (or adults) change their feelings in response to some external pressure, they usually do it in one of three ways:

1. Denial of feeling. Tim can tell himself that he is not feeling angry. He is not feeling anything at all.
2. Modifying the feeling. Tim can tell himself that it is not anger that he is feeling. It is something else.
3. Denial of responsibility. Tim can tell himself that it is not his fault that he is feeling angry. It is the fault of someone else. He is not responsible for how he feels. The process of blaming others reduces his power to make changes. If it is the fault of someone else, there is nothing he can do about it.

To broaden this concept, let us look at another example. Imagine Mary, a girl who is having problems learning in school. Her consistent failures are a source of fear and sadness for her. Her parents feel helpless and worried when confronted with her problems and her emotional reaction to them. They want to help her, but they don't know how. If they are not sensitive to her dilemma, they might react to their feelings of helplessness by communicating messages such as, "I am angry that you are not learning. You must not be trying hard enough."

Her teacher, fearing that perhaps her teaching methods are not adequate, might communicate messages such as, "I don't know what is wrong with you... Any normal child should be able to learn this... You are just not trying hard enough."

Mary might react to this situation in one of the three ways outlined above, denial of feeling, modifying the feeling, or denial of responsibility. She might take on attitudes such as:

"I am dumb. I am not normal. I am a failure."

"I don't care if I fail. I am not sad."

"I enjoy failing because it is a way of rebelling."

"It is not my fault that I am failing. It is the fault of someone else."

Peer pressure and bullying is another source of conflict for both adults and, especially, youngsters. It focuses attention on perceived shortcomings in areas like clothing, body type, weight, looks, and disabilities and places the victim in the situation of needing to find ways of thinking to diminish the pain of the experience.

These examples do not just apply to childhood. Adults use the same mechanisms to match their natural feelings to external expectations. Each time we do so, we forsake our inner self. Instead of acknowledging our feelings, accepting them, and allowing them to change naturally, we hide them, deny them, distort them, or refuse to accept responsibility for them.

If Mary were allowed to express her sadness and anger without blame or judgment, her feelings could serve as guides to point out where change is needed. She could begin to see how her needs and beliefs are creating her pain. She could begin to develop alternative perceptions of herself that would not rely upon external measures of success. She could begin to become aware of her inner goals for her life and trust her assessments of her progress toward these goals. Mary's feelings could also serve as an impetus for her teacher and parents to re-evaluate their expectations and the needs out of which these expectations grow.

Feelings are guides for change. When we block them, we stifle our growth and the growth of others around us. When we block our growth, we subject ourselves to a repetitive cycle of events in which those same feelings will be re-stimulated. Mary's failure will continue to be a source of pain for herself and her parents until they can recognize that external measures of success are unimportant; that such yardsticks have nothing to do with the worth of the person; and that, if anything, they are impediments to growth.

We should be striving for a clear channel through which all our true feelings may be acknowledged and expressed. If we have this clear channel, we can use our feelings to guide our growth. When your hand hurts, you know that it is time to take it off the hot stove. You do not demand that the stove become less hot so that you won't be hurt. You know that you must act to alleviate your pain. When we experience emotional pain, it should be telling us that change is needed and we should look within ourselves to see where the changes are required. This might involve changing the environment or relationships, but it is important to recognize that your mental structure has allowed that painful event to occur. It is your consciousness that must change in order to alleviate the pain.

Although change can bring uncertainty, fear, and anxiety, love, joy, and excitement are emotions that are stimulated when growth is taking place. These feelings are signs that positive changes are taking place in your mental structure. If we have a clear channel for our feelings, they can stimulate change, pass through us, and be gone. When we build dams across this channel the feelings can no longer pass by. They are held and begin to accumulate. They grow in energy and power and begin to seem stronger than ourselves. We begin to be frightened of losing control of them, for we do not know where they will take us. We might even begin to think that our feelings have a separate identity. We might feel that they are not part of ourselves, seeing them as coming from or belonging to those around us. We may then begin to fear a malevolent force. We see evil in ourselves and in the world around us. We begin to fear ourselves and to distrust our judgment. It then becomes necessary to seek outside of ourselves for knowledge. It becomes necessary to turn to gurus, churches, schools, political systems, and so forth to seek knowledge, reassurance, and forgiveness.

The most important message in this book is that the source of all knowledge lies within each and every one of us. Just as each individual cell within the body contains a complete knowledge of the entire body stored on its DNA molecules, so also does each of us contain a potential knowledge of God. Discovering our knowledge of God opens the path of joy and harmony. But this is not intellectual knowledge because our earthly concepts are incapable of describing what God is.

Each person is a part of God. Thinking of God is a mind-boggling task. The closest that I can come to conceptualizing it is to think that God is the sum total of all the energy that exists in the visible and invisible universes (matter being energy that is organized in a particular way so that we are able to perceive it). God is the perfect, loving energy that is the source of consciousness and all creation.

When God created the universe, it was a process whereby God encapsulated parts of His/Her energy and separated them from Him/Herself insofar as He/She gave the gift of self-determination to each of those energy capsules. Each energy capsule is a person who has total freedom of self-determination and yet is still a part of God. As such, each person is basically composed of that perfect, loving energy.

A parallel would be to think of each individual as being like a single cell in your body. Take a few moments to imagine what it would be like to be a cell. You would see yourself as a unique individual with distinct boundaries that separate you from all other cells. You would be surrounded by many other cells of varying shapes and sizes but all sharing similar functions and purposes. A sea of fluids around you would bring the nutrients that you need to survive, but you would have no idea where they came from. You would have been born from another cell and would anticipate a certain maximum life span. You would see other cells around you dying, with new cells being born to take their place. At various times, there would be hardships to deal with as toxic chemicals, viruses or bacteria enter your environment.

It would be very difficult to see that you are a part of an organ, although you might deduce that from the similarity of function of all your neighbors. It would be more difficult still to see that that organ is a part of a system that is part of a person. Even if you were aware that such a thing as a person existed, you would have no basis on which to understand the thoughts, feelings and purposes of that person.

And yet, within you, you would have the potential, coded on your DNA molecules, not only to understand that person but to reproduce that person. By looking around you, by studying your environment, it would be impossible to understand the person of whom you are a part. But, by looking within yourself, by studying the nature of your own being, you would have the capacity to understand that person.

Through creation, each of us was given the gift of creation. We became responsible for creating our experience. Even though we may not be aware of it, we are continually creating our inner conception of reality, as well as the potential for the events of our lives. God continually demonstrates His/Her love for us by supporting our creative process and supplying us with whatever experiences we choose to create, even when those experiences will bring us pain. Whatever we want to bring into our lives we will be permitted to experience.

The pathway that will lead us back to being that perfect, loving energy that is free from negativity, is the path of self-understanding. Nothing can force us in that direction or we would be giving up our free will. Only when we choose to expand our awareness can we see that we can take charge of our experience. When we are able to free ourselves from our negative thoughts and distorted feelings, we can begin to experience the joy of being in harmony with God.

All of our negative thoughts and feelings stem from the belief that someone or something else is in control of our lives. Fear, anger, sadness, and all their variants occur because we believe that someone or something else holds power over us—power to approve of us, to hurt us, to frustrate us, to deprive us, and so forth. When we realize that we hold these powers and no one else, we no longer need to experience emotions other than love and excitement.

Achieving the realization that each individual is his/her own creator enables one to see every person as being much like the sun on a cloudy day. The core is that capsule of perfect, loving energy, but it is covered by clouds of negative thoughts and feelings. We live in fear of each other's clouds and never see the sun that shines within each of us.

If you are able to accept that there is, within you, a core of that perfect, loving energy, you will have planted a seed that will begin to grow and, in growing, will begin to reveal the nature of the inner self. You can then begin to trust the guidance that is available through the inner self. This guidance is revealed through your intuition. It can provide the understanding that can lead you back to the love and perfection from which we all came.

The only positive actions that we can take are those that grow out of love. However, there can be no real love until there is self-acceptance. We cannot truly love until we are able to accept ourselves. The foundation of almost all psychological problems lies in the inability to accept aspects of oneself. When Freud talked about defense mechanisms, he was talking about ways in which we try to keep ourselves from consciously seeing who we are. Like Tim and Mary, cited in the earlier examples, we end up lying to ourselves about who we really are because we have learned to be ashamed or afraid of parts of ourselves. Concepts such as sin and karma make self-acceptance more difficult by reinforcing the idea that certain thoughts, feelings, and actions must be avoided.

I am not suggesting that we should all feel free to act as we wish. However, the task of achieving self-acceptance is made much more difficult when barriers are erected that stop us from exploring who we really are. The more we avoid thoughts and feelings the more frightening they become.

If I am unable to be honest with myself about my thoughts and feelings, I have no basis for change. How can I change if I do not know who I am? When I get down to really examining the thoughts and feelings that I fear, I find that I am surrounded by paper tigers. Those feelings only have power because I am afraid of them. As soon as I stop being afraid of them, they begin to change. When I stop being afraid of my feelings, I stop being afraid of other people. When I am able to accept myself, I am able to accept others for who they are. When I am able to get past the barriers of fear, rigidity, needs, and guilt, when I get down to what is underneath it all, I find that there is love and acceptance that flows easily because it is the basic energy that we are all made of. If I can accept my negative feelings, I can give them up and become part of universal love.

In order to facilitate greater self-acceptance, I would recommend the following exercise: Three times a day, for two weeks, write the following statement five times at each sitting. "I am (your first name). My existence is important. I am a creation of love and am learning to be my own creator."

I would also recommend the practice of meditation. Here are some basic guidelines:

1. Choose a time and place where you will not be disturbed.
2. Depending on your age and flexibility, select a posture that best suits you. The most important aspect of posture is an erect spine (allowing easy flow of breath). This can range from a full lotus position to sitting on a gomden, to sitting in a chair.
3. Set a timer that will define the length of your meditation session. I would recommend 15–30 minutes. Do not end the meditation session before the timer signals the end of the session, no matter how much your mind tells you that you have better things to do.
4. As you sit in meditation, focus on your breath. This can be done by imagining breathing in one nostril and out the other or by visualizing a balloon that swells with the in-breath and deflates with the out-breath. Inflate your lungs fully and exhale completely.
5. As thoughts emerge, do not dwell on them. Acknowledge that you are thinking and let the thoughts go. This applies to all nagging thoughts, emotions, inspirations, and so on. Go back to focusing on the breath and let the thoughts go.

If you follow the foregoing recommendations, you will probably find that your mind will not leave you alone. Thoughts will constantly intrude and it will be easy to get involved in those thoughts. It will take a great deal of practice before you will be able to experience moments of clear consciousness that are free from worries, hopes, fears, anger, and so on. I would recommend doing meditation practice daily and persisting over months or years.

Chapter 4
Experience

A term such as experience is difficult to define in a discrete way. We all know what it is to have experienced something, but it would be almost impossible to define the limits of a single experience or event. All the events of our lives blend into each other and become interdependent in such a way that it is difficult to see where one begins and another ends. The events of the present often have roots deep within our past. The choices we make today are serving to shape the events of the future.

For this reason, the term experience will remain very loosely defined throughout the material that follows. It can be thought of as being our perception of the interrelated sequence of events that fill our life space.

Our experience is the medium through which the process of personal growth can take place. It is also an expression of our consciousness. Since our experience is shaped by our needs, values, and beliefs, the events of our lives truly are an expression of the mental structure we have constructed. So, at once, our experience is both our creative product and our medium for further creative change.

Life provides us with experience and thus with the opportunity to create changes within ourselves. This is what existence in the material world offers us. It provides us with a mirror of our consciousness. Our mental structure is expressed in a way that provides us with the opportunity to view it as though it were not part of us. Our consciousness becomes expressed as life events.

For example, a lack of self-acceptance may be expressed as an abusive parent, spouse, or friend; a belief in the need to control others may result in a position of power and influence; a belief in the wickedness of others may find expression in being the victim of their crimes; and a belief in the basic goodness of one's fellow man may result in experiencing acts of kindness and understanding.

Our life in the material world is somewhat like being attached to a biofeedback machine. Our mental structure is constantly being reflected back to us through the events of our lives. When we wish to make changes, we have a concrete medium within which to work. Without our existence in this reality, we would be in a position like someone who had learned the theory of how to drive, but who had never been in a car. Physical existence gives us the chance to allow new learning to be an integral part of our being, just as the mechanics of driving become second nature to the experienced motorist. We are here to learn and to grow and this takes place through our experience.

We grow most of all when we take responsibility for our experiences. If we recognize that everything that happens in our lives is a reflection of the mental structure which we have constructed then we are in a position to use experiences effectively. No one is responsible for the happiness of another person. We may choose to believe that we are responsible for others or that they are responsible for us, but, in the final analysis, the ultimate responsibility lies with the individual himself. When we find ourselves entangled in the problems of others, it is because we have involved ourselves. Granted, we may be able to justify our involvement through our mental structure of values, needs, and beliefs, but without this mental structure, the entanglements are illusory. This is especially apparent when you examine human behavior across various cultures.

What is perfectly logical and necessary behavior in one culture will make no sense at all in another culture. It is the depth of our commitment to our values and beliefs that leaves us blind to the fact that we do have choices in every situation we encounter. Whenever we feel that we have no choice about our behavior, it is because we are not allowing ourselves to explore our beliefs.

But what about the circumstances of our birth and our childhood? What of illnesses and other disasters that might befall us in our lifetime? Are these also of our own choosing?

To argue these points is an interesting exercise in creative thinking. I tend to believe that such factors are also a part of the mirror image of our consciousness that life provides for us. I feel that the circumstances of our birth are a projection of the type of learning that we most need to experience. We are provided with circumstances that are most likely to lead to growth in the areas we most need.

With respect to health, it is becoming more and more evident that our health is an extension of our state of mind. The body responds in ways that we are only just beginning to understand the mental and emotional state of the individual. Our consciousness plays a big role in determining our health. Our health is also like a feedback system to let us know when we are on the wrong track. If we would learn to listen to the wisdom of our bodies we would discover a guide who is well prepared to assist us on the pathway to growth.

Fortunately, it is not necessary to resolve these arguments in order to adopt an attitude that will permit us to get the most out of all our experiences. That attitude is to say to yourself, "I am going to treat every circumstance and every experience in my life as a unique opportunity to learn more about myself and to change myself in accordance with my learning." What is initially seen as misfortune can be a blessing in disguise. It may shake us out of a rut that was leading nowhere. It may force us to make changes in ourselves that we may have otherwise avoided. It may change our direction in life in important ways that we may only recognize years later. It may provide us with unique opportunities for learning that we might never have otherwise had. It may create strengths that we might never have otherwise developed. All of these things are possible if we remain open-minded and determined to make the most of all our experiences.

Take a few minutes to think back over your life. When did the greatest learning and personal growth take place? Was it in times of tranquility and security or was it during times of uncertainty and adjustment? The willingness to accept total responsibility for your life sets the stage for real growth to begin to take place.

You Are Your Own Creator

When you can acknowledge the truth in this statement, you begin to assume control over your life which you may never have experienced before. You are giving up your excuses. You can no longer blame others for the events of your life. In return, you will receive a sense of freedom that you will not have had before. Your life is your responsibility. You can make it into what you want. You have only yourself to answer to. Others have control over you only if you give it to them.

The suggestion of such responsibility may create anxiety for many people. We have all been conditioned to believe that if we are not controlled by others, we will become immoral and irresponsible. Greed, hatred, lust, and jealousy are presumed to be natural human qualities that, if unchecked, will inevitably lead to antisocial behavior. Frankly, I find such thinking unacceptable. I believe very strongly in the need for growth as the basic human striving. When growth is taking place, the individual naturally experiences feelings of love, joy, and excitement. When growth is consistently blocked through distorted needs, values, and beliefs, these positive emotions can become transmuted into greed, hatred, lust, and jealousy. However, these do not represent the basic human condition.

Ask yourself whether you want to bring harm to others. If you do not wish to harm others, then you will take care of their needs and feelings. If you do wish to harm others, then you would be well advised to seek out someone who can help you understand yourself better.

Remember that your mental structure, that is your beliefs, values, and needs, is the mechanism through which your experiences are interpreted and made meaningful or meaningless.

Remember also that this mental structure is totally subject to change. There is nothing absolute in your mental structure any more than there is anything absolute in our material universe.

Recent developments in theoretical physics are leading to the thesis that there is nothing concrete or real other than energy, which is organized in special ways. Einstein demonstrated that time is relative to the viewer and that it can be slowed and even stopped. Time is an abstract concept that we use to account for changes in our perceptions. Physicists have demonstrated that matter can be changed into energy. As they examine smaller and smaller particles, they discover that matter is energy. Physical objects are ninety-nine percent empty space. The particles that do exist are actually energy forms composed of one single type of energy.

If this is the case, then our physical world truly is an illusion. So also is our mental structure an illusion of a reality that exists because we create it. However, this is in no way to suggest that it is all meaningless.

On the contrary, it opens the door to a profound meaningfulness in life. Life becomes the stage about which Shakespeare wrote, but each of us is our own director. We can begin to see our lives in perspective. We are not the parts we play. We are more than that. The different parts are only opportunities to learn different things about ourselves. The mental structure we hold is only one possible way of perceiving our experience. If your learning had been different, if you were raised in a different culture or by different parents, your needs, values, and beliefs would have been different. A different mental structure would give you a different view of your experiences. What a wonderfully diverse place this world is when viewed in that way.

As you begin to allow changes in your mental structure, your view of your experiences will change. You may begin to sense the creative potential that exists in this area. Experiences can become your tools rather than your master. The exercises in the chapters that follow will give you guidelines to help you establish a greater awareness and sense of control over your mental structure.

I would like to suggest that you think of experiences as the fifth dimension. Events take place in space which is defined by the three dimensions of length, width, and height. They also are perceived to occur in a temporal sequence which is defined by the fourth dimension of time. In addition, there is a quality of meaningfulness and intensity of perception which takes us into the fifth dimension of experience. This fifth dimension affects our perception of time, allowing us to perceive it as moving very slowly or very quickly. It allows events to be perceived with intensity and meaningfulness, or to pass practically unnoticed. It is a measure of the richness and beauty of our perception of events.

The richness of our perceptions is determined to a large extent by the number of different aspects we can perceive in a particular event. Meaningfulness is enriched when we are able to apply many different interpretations to an event.

To better understand this, try to visualize an event as a many-sided surface such as a cube. Each surface represents a different aspect of that experience, a different way of interpreting that experience. For example, consider the experience of a young person moving away from his parent's home. The many surfaces of this event might include such aspects as:

a. it will enable the person to learn personal responsibility;

b. it may give the chance to find new sources of love;

c. it may provide new avenues for creativity;

d. it may open up new sources of friendship;

e. these new experiences may allow for a greater sense of self-worth;

f. it will allow the person the opportunity to develop their own values;

g. it is an opportunity for increasing self-knowledge.

The accompanying diagram illustrates how this experience can be viewed in different ways. Each different perspective will offer different learning to the viewer. Different viewers may experience totally different learning. Yet all the learning is contained in the same experience. What we gain from a particular experience at a particular time very much depends upon who we are and what we are looking for at that time.

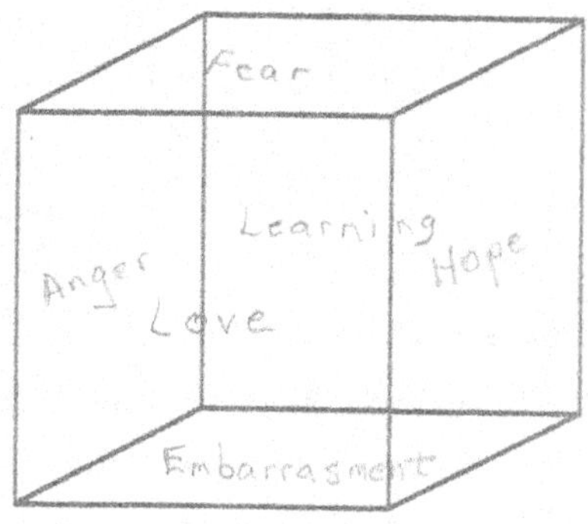

Another example of the multifaceted quality of experience is to consider the multitude of motivations that people have for going to parties. Thinking of a party as a single event or experience, one is able to see the many different facets of this polyhedron. Making new friends, seeking recognition or approval from others, releasing tension, finding a sexual partner, escaping from boredom, seeking intellectual stimulation, strengthening existing relationships with friends, putting in an appearance to avoid hurting the feelings of others, getting drunk or stoned, an opportunity to make an impression on someone, facilitating a business deal—each of these might form a different aspect of the experience. Which aspect you focus on will determine what you get out of the experience.

If you think about our collective lives, there really is not a great deal of variability in our experiences. But, if you consider the many aspects of each experience, you can see that there really does not need to be. So many different perspectives and opportunities for learning can be extracted from an event that we can re-use the same events over and over and each time extract some new learning from them. What we learn from the events of our lives varies according to what our needs and thoughts are at the time they occur. How you use an experience then really depends upon which aspect or aspects you are looking at. The more surfaces you are able to perceive in an experience the more you are able to savor that experience as a real opportunity for learning. If, however, you always focus on only one aspect of an experience, little growth takes place.

When people have very strong needs or high degrees of fear or anxiety, they often tend to focus on the same surface in all experiences and reject experiences that do not offer that surface. Imagine, for example, the effect on the experiences in one's life if a person becomes strongly fixated on the need for self-esteem, security, or sexual expression, or any other single aspect of events. It is not difficult to see where they would be placing great limits on their learning.

Seeking out and being open to new aspects of experiences can make otherwise mundane experiences meaningful and meaningful experiences much more so. Now, as an exercise, think of a recent event in your life. Write down as many potential aspects of this experience as you can think of. Find at least one new aspect which you have not previously considered. Repeat this process by looking at some other events of your life. Work toward building the habit of looking at all sides of the events of your life. Try to see some new opportunities for learning in each experience you examine.

In all of our experiences, we are continuously making choices. At any given moment, we have an almost infinite number of choices available to us as to what we will do next. We also have a choice as to what aspects of our experiences we will look at. Frequently, however, we feel that we have no choice, but to go on making the same choices as we always have. Some of these choices grow out of habits that we may be unaware of or that we tell ourselves we are unable to change. Some choices are made as being the safest path, the one that will result in the least anxiety, insecurity, or pain. Until we are able to take responsibility for the fact that we are making choices, it becomes very difficult to make changes in our actions and perceptions.

In order to get a better sense of how you are shaping your life through your choices, try taking a day or a part of a day and clarifying your choices by stating them to yourself. For example, you may get up in the morning by saying, "I choose to get up now. All things considered, it is what I most want to do," rather than saying, "I have to get up now." Continue making statements about your choices throughout the day.

"I choose to snap at the children. It is what I most want to do."

"I choose to have a cigarette. I can quit, but I choose not to."

"I choose not to go to the museum, library, park, tennis courts, or movies today. All things considered, I would rather go to work."

"I choose not to talk to the people in the elevator this morning. I know that it is possible to make the world a friendlier place by putting out a little friendliness myself, but I choose not to do that."

So often we feel like victims of our life circumstances. When we do so, we forsake the element of choice. We feel helpless to be able to change the things that happen in our lives or the way that we feel about them. This feeling is also a choice we have made. Whenever I feel trapped, I know that my needs, beliefs, and, values are serving to close off all my choices. I must then remind myself that those needs, beliefs, and values are of my choosing and that I may change them if I wish. A re-evaluation of my mental structure is required if I wish to have greater choice. Growth must take place. That feeling of being trapped becomes an opportunity for personal growth in order to move past it.

Remember that who you are now is a summation of all the choices you have made in your life up to this point. You cannot look at your present circumstances and how they trap you without looking at the choices you have made to bring you to where you are now. In looking at all those past choices you should be able to recognize the needs, beliefs, and feelings on which those choices were based. If you can admit these things to yourself honestly, it should give you material with which to formulate a new definition of yourself.

As an exercise to expand your awareness in this area, take a particular experience in your life and look at it from different perspectives. First of all, consider how you first interpreted it. The interpretation might have been positive or negative. Then think of the experience from a different perspective. As an example, I think of when my grade 9 yearbook came out in our school. I was a very anxious person and generally expected a negative reaction from other people. The caption under my picture said, 'The face we like to see'. I immediately interpreted this in a negative way. I thought that it was being suggested that I was cutting classes, which was something that I never did. I was confused and upset by the caption. It was only years later that it occurred to me that it might have been referring to the fact that I was relatively good-looking. If I had interpreted it in this way at the time, it might have resulted in me relaxing some of my anxiety about how others viewed me and might have resulted in me being more open to others.

There are many different experiences that one might examine in this way. Some might be experiences that were upsetting at the time. For example, something that someone said that was distressing or a disappointing outcome for something you were hoping to achieve. It might have something to do with your life circumstances, such as family problems or the failure of a relationship. It might also be something that you viewed as positive, such as winning a competition. Look at the event in as many ways as you can, considering how your interpretation affected your life or the lives of others and how an alternative point of view might have had different consequences. Interpreting those events in a different way can still change the ultimate consequences of the event.

Chapter 5
Wants, Needs, Desires

Wants, needs, desires, and dreams all fall in the general category of motivation. Motivation is critical in understanding behavior. It is like the engine of your psyche. Just like in an automobile, the engine moves the car, but it is the driver that determines the direction it takes. If you, the reader, are seeking to understand yourself and to make changes, it is important to understand what motivates you and how you direct your motivation. I would first like to discuss needs. These fall into three general categories: physical needs, needs for safety, and psychological/emotional needs.

Physical needs

The physical needs are the most obvious of all the needs. Without a doubt, we need food, water, air, sleep, and warmth. Without these, life cannot go on. Many people have these needs met adequately, but there are those for whom life is a struggle for existence. While this forms the basis for their daily lives, they still have psychological and emotional needs.

Research on maternal deprivation has suggested that infants have a strong need for gentle physical contact. It is evident even among animals that they will seek out close contact with other animals. Sometimes this even happens with members of another species. (Think about those cute UTube videos about strange relationships among animals.) Bowlby, the first researcher to focus on the effect of disrupting the relationship of a child with his/her primary parenting figure (assumed in his era, the 1950s, to be the mother), observed that children brought up in an environment lacking in physical nurturing, such as orphanages, resulted in children who lacked emotional depth and who had a greater incidence of emotional and behavioral problems.

Also, in the 1950s, Harlow carried out research on rhesus monkeys who were deprived of any contact with a living mother. He found that it resulted in major distortions in social and sexual behaviors. This information suggests that there is a fundamental need for love and physical contact with others. The need for physical contact can become sexualized in puberty and through adulthood.

Physical needs have a powerful effect on the mind. I first learned this when I attempted to quit smoking. I would start out with the best intentions, determined to follow through. As the desire for nicotine increased, however, my thinking would change. Thoughts would emerge rationalizing that it was okay to smoke and I would give in. When I did quit, it took strong determination to resist the rationalizations. I am sure that anyone who has tried dieting has probably experienced the same thing. The physical desire alters your thinking to justify why it is okay to give in…just this time.

I observed the same thing when working with sex offenders in a forensic setting. Many of them felt badly about what they did. When we would examine their actions, it was apparent that the offense would start with an aberrant thought that would be kept secret from others. The thought might not have involved any intention at first. As sexual desire increased, the thought grew stronger and stronger and rationalizations started to creep in. Since the person did not talk to anyone about the thoughts and feelings they were having, there was no corrective feedback. Eventually, the desire and its rationalizations would be strong enough to lead to action and the offense was committed.

The moral of what I am saying is to be aware of your physical needs and how they might impact your behavior. The reason that support groups, such as Alcoholics Anonymous, Narcotics Anonymous, Sexaholics Anonymous, and dieting clubs, are important is that they provide a venue for talking about distorted thoughts and feelings and getting support and feedback from others.

Fear and safety

According to the theory of Abraham Maslow, a personality theorist, needs fall into a hierarchy that determines what needs are more primary. He placed physical needs as being first in terms of importance. He believed that the need for safety was next in order of importance. Safety can be thought of as the need to preserve one's physical integrity, but it can also be manifest as need for security of finances, relationships, and so on.

It has been suggested that we live in a fear-based reality. By that, I mean that the underlying motivation for many human behaviors is fear. We do not like uncertainty and we are inclined to think in a persevering fashion about negative outcomes. One of the biggest challenges in personal growth is to let go of fear and live life as it unfolds. Life is bound to hold some unpleasant experiences. It cannot be avoided. What I do know, though, is that the fear of what might happen is ultimately more painful than the actual events. I have many times anticipated that this or that event is going to be unpleasant or difficult, only to find that it was not nearly as bad as I thought. And when events are truly painful and difficult, they often come unexpectedly.

I am not trying to suggest that people do not sometimes find themselves in consistently painful circumstances. Victims of family violence, sexual abuse, bullying, brutality, and torture experience great emotional and physical pain, but the anticipation and fear of the pain create as much emotional distress as the pain itself. When painful circumstances are actually occurring, we are generally preoccupied with coping and finding ways of managing the situation and this reduces the pain we are experiencing.

In summary, I would say that one should strive to be free of negative expectations and to allow experiences to unfold without anticipation. Being in the moment is the best preparation for whatever will come your way. Being in the moment also allows you to tap into levels of consciousness beyond emotion that may offer more productive outcomes to the dilemma.

Psychological needs

Human beings are social animals and the need to be loved and to belong is very important. I have mentioned the need for love under physical needs because the failure to experience love can have devastating results physically and emotionally. Children who come from loving, supportive families generally thrive, while children who have been neglected struggle. Since one cannot make others love you, the important thing is to be receptive to love. Negative thoughts, feelings, and behaviors, such as fear, distrust, competitiveness, and withdrawal, can stand in the way of establishing relationships that might provide love and a sense of belonging. It is necessary to set aside these barriers by being aware of them and by letting down one's guard.

Self-esteem has been identified as a psychological need, but this needs some interpretation. Self-esteem implies that one should think of themselves in a positive manner. Doing so involves comparing oneself to others in order to find ways in which you stand equal to or above them. I would suggest that we should instead strive to have a neutral view of ourselves. Each of us has our talents, but we are not greater or lesser than others. True self-esteem does not require reassurance. True self-esteem involves living life in a thoughtful way that is in accord with inner values, moment by moment doing what is right, and having no regrets about how your life has unfolded. True self-esteem involves being open and receptive and being willing to alter one's thoughts and values when it is evident that change is required. Criticism can be tolerated and made use of when it is constructive. True self-esteem does not cling to a self-image and allows new thoughts and feelings to emerge.

There is a category of psychological needs that has been termed self-actualization needs. These are needs that involve creative impulses. We have a need to create something (e.g., painting, pottery, woodwork, needlework, poetry, writing), not because we need these things, but because it fulfills a need for artistic expression. Art can communicate things that cannot easily be put into words. Some people express these needs in a more physical way, such as mountain climbing, scuba diving, gymnastics, skiing, sports, and so on. These activities set challenges that are achieved solely for the purpose of knowing that you can do them. Self-actualization can also be expressed in helping relationships where the motive truly is to be of benefit to another person in their life journey. Self-actualization grows out of inspiration and creative expression where the action is its own reward and there is no strong need for recognition or acknowledgment.

Wants

In a consumer society, wants can be a strong motivating factor in behavior. We are confronted with a wide array of things that we might possess and we are subject to pressures like advertising, keeping up with the Joneses, peer pressure, status, and prestige, and so on. Wants run through all socio-economic levels of society. Poor children might dream about having the designer clothes that their peers wear or be distressed about being the only one in their group without a smartphone. Poor parents might want better accommodation, a bed that does not sag, or a roof that does not leak.

Middle-class people might be looking for a better car, a lawn mower, a dishwasher, or a bigger house. Wealthy people might think about belonging to a prestigious golf club, having a large yacht, or being able to throw lavish parties. It seems that the wants never end. Once one thing is possessed, it loses its significance and a new want replaces it. Wants are part of life, but they have very little to do with spiritual growth or self-development, particularly once people are beyond the subsistence level. The fulfillment of wants can give the illusion that one is progressing in life but this is an empty process.

Steering the Ship

Needs are an important aspect of our mental structure. They guide our behavior. They are the motivation that leads to action on our part. They are, in large part, responsible for determining which side of the cube we look at in our experiences. They draw certain aspects of experience into focus while closing off other aspects and other experiences. In almost every action we are expressing a need, although we do not necessarily think of the need in a conscious fashion.

"This is what I am meant to do." One often hears this statement or something similar. It is an interesting statement insofar as what it implies. The implication is that there is a guiding hand in our lives that is of God-like proportions and that our lives have a predestined quality. But how do we distinguish what is predestined from what we hope or desire? I do not want to argue whether there is a greater plan for our lives or whether our lives are simply the product of our efforts. If all is predestined, then we are likely to arrive at our destination regardless of what we do.

There are occasions in all of our lives where we can see that fate or luck has brought us to a certain place. There are some strange coincidences that periodically have a significant influence on the circumstances that we end up in. This can be for the better or for the worse (judged on the basis of what we want). It might be the accidental meeting of someone who will come to be an important person in our lives or it could be an accumulation of circumstances that allow us to achieve or prevent us from achieving something that we are working toward or that we desire. For example, think of the number of people whose lives have been altered by war, famine, illness, accident, poverty, social disruption, or the death of someone whom they are close to.

In the Western world, we tend to think that obstacles can be heroically overcome, but sometimes the frustration of our efforts can, in the long run, be for the better. When you think back to times when things did not work out as you hoped, can you see that it was because there was an opportunity for something more fulfilling? But there are also times when circumstances have led to what seems to be a mundane life. Women are often faced with difficult choices about pursuing occupational goals or giving their efforts to children and families.

How do we know what is truly (from a divine predestination perspective) intended for our lives? We tend to look to societal values in determining the worth of our lives. Those outcomes that are seen as most meritorious and that would bring us the greatest public adulation are what we tend to see as desirable. A career as a singer that brings fame and glory is more coveted than using one's voice to soothe and entertain friends and family members. A career as a doctor or lawyer is seen as desirable regardless of how well that suits the character of the person.

How can we know what we are intended to do? Or are we intended to do anything in particular? It might be useful to look at the collective of humanity in thinking of our intended purpose. There are so many different cultures and values. What might be considered important in one culture might not be considered as such in another. And yet there are commonalities in all cultures.

Humanistic values are pretty well universal. Caring for one's children in a loving and nurturing way, being a loyal friend, not causing harm to others, being generous, and contributing to the general well-being of the community are the types of values that are seen as important throughout the world. Some of the most significant acts are ones that are never acknowledged.

It seems that there is a persistent struggle between acts that are founded in love and acts that are founded in the seven deadly sins: pride, greed, lust, envy, gluttony, wrath, and sloth. With a few exceptions, it seems that the higher up the societal power hierarchy one looks, the more likely it is that actions are motivated by the latter. What we are exposed to in the media is often related to the seven deadly sins and the exercise of power. Fame is valued, as is wealth and influence.

If we are looking for what is intended for our lives, it is easy to get lost in what is portrayed, directly or indirectly, as desirable. And yet the daily functioning of the world is most strongly dependent on the small acts of unknown individuals: store clerks, mothers, tradesmen, medical personnel, and so forth. We could more easily do without a famous singer, actor, or politician than we could do without someone to nurture our children or unplug our toilet.

One might suggest that the purpose of humanity is to eventually become a cohesive entity in which love is the guiding principle. That would suggest that the purpose of each individual is to contribute to that ultimate goal. When looking at the world from the perspective of power and control, it is discouraging to think that this ultimate purpose could ever be achieved, but when you look around at the seemingly insignificant people in the world, there is much more reason to hope. Some of the most thoughtful and generous people are those who have the least to give.

If we are looking for divine direction or spiritual guidance, it would be best to focus on living our lives guided by love and concern for others. Instead of the seven deadly sins, we could strive for humility, generosity, temperance, goodwill, moderation, forgiveness, encouragement, and diligence. The road of your life will lead somewhere. You will be able to hold the reins and give it a nudge, but bear in mind that where you think you are going might not be what is intended. Be open. Let life guide you.

So let us now extend the definition of our needs beyond those physical and material needs. The needs that are, by far, the most important in determining our growth are those that focus on social, psychological, and spiritual aspects of ourselves. If we tell ourselves that we need a large quantity of material things, our behavior will become strongly oriented toward obtaining those things. We will take on extra work, work longer hours, and become more interested in finding ways to make money to obtain the things that we want. It is a basic law of behavior that the stronger the incentive, the greater the motivation. The greater the motivation, the longer and harder the individual will strive for the goal.

It is most logical to consider the same to be true of social, psychological, and spiritual needs. The more clearly we define an aspect of our experience as a need and the more we see that need to be important, the harder we will strive to fill that need. One of the big obstacles we have to overcome in this regard is that, in general, we are not encouraged to think about these categories of needs. The material aspects of our existence are more clearly seen as involving needs than are the mental and emotional ones. Consequently, people are very often unaware of what motivates their behavior in relation to themselves and others.

When the individual lacks an awareness of his own unique and personal needs, it is unlikely that those needs will be filled in any meaningful way. In such a situation we end up playing a role. We do what we think is expected of us without any real consideration of our uniqueness. We end up living our lives according to the expectations of others. The true self is not allowed expression and, consequently, has no opportunity to develop. We begin to stagnate and to waste the precious opportunity that life affords us.

Unless you are able to recognize and acknowledge a need, it is unlikely that the need will ever really be filled, even though your experiences may provide many opportunities for fulfillment. As was described earlier, what experience you take out of an event depends upon which aspect of the event you focus on. Your needs direct this process. You will find a need being filled only if you look for the fulfillment of that need in your experiences.

A good illustration of this can be found by comparing some of your moments of depression with times when you are feeling emotionally high. As a rule, depression is accompanied by a negative attitude in which nothing seems to be very satisfying. Although we might be looking for love or self-esteem, none of the events that occur during the depression seem to offer such possibilities. However, if the same events were to occur during an emotional high, we are likely to find these needs easily met. As with the Biblical phrase, "Seek and ye shall find," it seems to be necessary to define the need before it can be filled, to formulate the question before it can be answered.

The growth of self-understanding is a step-by-step process. As each need is met, a new need arises which leads to higher levels of understanding. Each need prepares us for new learning. It will present an opportunity to look at new aspects of ourselves. The questions that are formed in relation to each need are vital in expanding our understanding. The questioning process allows for movement beyond the current need.

As in science, the questions that you ask yourself are the keys to growth. Every scientific advance has come as a result of someone asking the right question. The answers usually take care of themselves. They are frequently obvious when the right questions are asked. The fulfillment of a need is like priming a pump. It is a necessary condition for growth but will not, in itself, produce growth. Questioning the need allows for movement into new areas of understanding.

There are several potential problems that may interfere with the effective utilization of needs to direct our growth. The first has already been discussed. If you do not have an awareness of your needs, growth will be very difficult to achieve. I am afraid that this is, all too often, the human condition. Each of us is exposed to influences from a variety of sources that may direct the needs that we focus on. To some extent, we choose to listen to those influences that coincide with our needs. However, these influences may also direct us into areas that do not coincide with the needs of the inner self.

I would like to illustrate this with a personal example. Clinical psychology can be a very emotionally demanding job, especially if you have unresolved needs or conflicts that are brought out by your clients' problems. This was my experience for most of my early years in the profession. I was trying very hard to do the best I knew how for my clients, but it was emotionally exhausting. I felt that there must be a career that was better suited to my needs.

After discussing the matter with my wife, I decided that I would seek acceptance in medical school. Medicine, as a career, offered everything that our society told me that I should need. It offered money, prestige, and freedom. I knew that my family would be pleased with such a success. If I could accomplish this, I would have everything I believed I needed. The odds were against me because of my age and my lack of a science background. However, I worked hard. I committed myself to the task of being accepted into a program. A year later, I had what I wanted. I was accepted into a program.

By this time, however, I was beginning to realize that becoming a physician was not what I needed. I was starting to recognize that society's values did not reflect my needs. We had never lived in such a way that we really needed a great deal of money. I began to see that the recognition and prestige that I sought was only a poor substitute for a genuine feeling of self-acceptance. I needed someone else to say I was important because I did not really believe that I was. I knew that the freedom I was seeking was something that could only come from overcoming my fears and growing beyond my perceived needs. Now I can see that going to medical school would have been a terrible mistake. If I had, I would have made a very large commitment to needs that were not a reflection of my inner self. When I decided not to go, I decided to seek the path that was based on the needs of my inner self, even though I had no idea where that would lead me. Ultimately, it led to obtaining a Ph.D. in clinical neuropsychology and a lengthy, satisfying, and fulfilling career.

A second block to the effective utilization of needs is when we attempt to define how our needs will be met. This is particularly true in close personal relationships, such as with our parents or our children. I think most of us would have to admit that, at one time or another, we have needed our parents, children, or spouse to be someone different than who they really are in order to meet our own needs. I would again like to illustrate this with a personal example.

As a young person, I had difficulty forming any close friendships and frequently chose to feel isolated and rejected in my peer group. There were a number of painful memories associated with this pattern and the pattern continued into my adult life. I had a strong need to achieve self-acceptance and this was reflected in my need for approval from those around me. I also needed my wife and children to be approved of by others. When they were not, I needed them to change their behavior so that they would be. I can still remember the emotional anguish I experienced one day when our daughter was snubbed by a friend. I needed her not to feel the things I had felt as a child.

The more we need someone to be different than they are, the more we drive a wedge into the relationship. The more we demand of others, the further we push them away. I now recognize that real love is based on acceptance. You truly love someone when you do not need them to be any different than they are when you do not need anything from that other person, but you still choose to be with them. When you demand that your needs must be filled in certain ways, you close yourself off from the experience of love.

A third area of difficulty occurs when values close off certain needs. I think this is well illustrated in the area of self-acceptance. The concept of original sin that is contained in the Christian religion promotes the idea that we should avoid pride in ourselves, be self-abasing, and be aware of our basically wicked and sinful nature. Such values conflict with the need for self-acceptance. I have frequently discussed the need for self-acceptance and a sense of self-worth with groups. In these discussions, it has been the rare person who has admitted to liking themselves.

Most of us have been conditioned to believe that it is somehow wrong to like ourselves. We make constant comparisons with others and social media has only made this tendency worse.

If you can believe that your needs will be met and if you are vigilant to see how the events of your life are presenting experiences that will meet them, you can begin to see that you do live in a world of abundance. The needs that you focus on will be met when they are a true expression of the inner self, although they may not be met in the way that you expect them to be. Recognize that your basic needs are very simple. Question the needs you feel that you have and look for the simple needs that underlie them. Be flexible and recognize that events will be created that will allow your needs to be met.

When those simple needs are met, you will be able to experience true freedom. That is the freedom of having no urgent needs, of experiencing events without requiring anything from them. You will be able to experience the joy of pure being, moment by moment without the need for the past or the future.

There are two very simple exercises that can be used to develop a deeper level of awareness and understanding of your own personal needs and the impact they are having on your life. The first should give you an idea of your current level of awareness of your needs. It involves listing the needs that are a part of your present reality. Write down as many as you can possibly think of, whether they are large or small. Do not criticize any ideas that come to mind. If you think of something as a need, write it down. Remember, you are attempting to understand what motivates your behavior now as well as to gain a greater awareness of unexpressed aspects of yourself. Do not limit yourself to material things. In fact, the exercise will be most helpful if you focus on your social, psychological, and spiritual needs.

I have used this exercise a number of times with groups and with individuals. Frequently, it is found to be a very difficult exercise to do. Some people are unable to think of a single thing to write down. This is usually true for people who place the needs of others ahead of their own. In particular, women and, especially, mothers may have to work harder to discover what their needs are. Although this may seem noble, it presents some real barriers to personal growth. No matter how much you may wish to care for others, that desire is founded on personal needs that must be acknowledged if growth is to take place. Do not be discouraged if you draw a blank on this exercise. Continue to work on this area until you start to develop a free flow of ideas as to what your needs are. The next exercise will be of further assistance.

When you have completed your list, you should have a fairly good idea of your current level of awareness of your needs. You may have had little difficulty in completing the list. If this is the case, you may be prepared to begin working on another area. Before you do, however, there are a few questions you should ask yourself. Try to answer them as honestly as possible.

Are the needs that you have listed truly an expression of your inner self or are they things that you have come to believe that you need because of some outside influence such as parents, school, television, or your contemporaries?

Are these needs related to your personal growth? If they were fulfilled, would they contribute to your becoming a more loving and understanding person toward yourself and others?

Do these needs focus on your own personal responsibility for your experience or do they put the onus on someone else to fulfill your needs?

Listed below are some examples of needs as expressed from these two points of view.

Personal Responsibility	Responsibility to Others
"I need to free myself from the feeling of being dominated by others."	"I need my spouse to stop telling me what to do."
"I need to learn how I am closing myself off from love."	"I need someone to love me."
"I need to understand my feelings about certain relationships in my life."	"I need people to act differently toward me."

This is an important point to understand. Remember, you are the creator of your own experience. The people who are a part of your life and your relationships with them are an expression of your own consciousness. They reflect the degree of understanding that you have of yourself in various areas. As your understanding of yourself grows, your relationships with those people will change. If you focus on trying to change others into what you want them to be, you will have a very difficult task because you are ignoring the fact that you have, through your mental structure, created that relationship. If you can understand how you are creating it, then you can change it by changing some of your needs and beliefs.

If you do not feel that you have as much awareness of your needs as you would like to have, the next exercise will help to expand your definition of what your needs are and give you further awareness of your needs.

For a period of time (a day, a few days, a week) no matter what you find yourself doing, make the statement to yourself, "I need to…" and complete it with whatever you are doing at that time. For example, "I need to watch television."

"I need to read this book."

"I need to be in bed."

"I need to sit and do nothing."

Then begin to expand this process to include a greater range of your social and psychological behavior. Your statements might begin to sound like, "I need to be tense when I am talking to others."

"I need to be understood by someone."

"I need to have the attention of someone."

"I need to be loved."

"I need to love and respect myself."

Of course, many of the statements you make will sound untrue or ridiculous. But, if they do, this should be a signal to you. If you do not need to be doing, thinking, or feeling that, then why are you? Are you acting on the basis of your own unique inner needs, or are you allowing your need to please others to blind you to yourself?

As you begin to identify needs, no matter how small, write them down. Expand your list as your awareness grows. Go through the questions listed earlier in order to identify important areas for your personal growth.

An awareness of your needs is a basic building block in the growth process. Without it, your efforts will be wasted. It will be like planning a meal without knowing who will be eating it or building a house without knowing who will live in it. The extent to which the activities of your life create opportunities for your development will depend on your awareness of your needs. The effort you expend in this area will be well worthwhile. Do not leave this task until you are able to freely list your needs without hesitation or uncertainty. You should be able to confidently identify the needs that are truly an expression of your inner self and not just the fulfillment of a role or expectation. You should know when you are taking responsibility for your needs and when you are trying to pass the responsibility off to others. When you have accomplished this, you will be in a position to know what will lead to inner growth for you. It has been said that one should 'choose the path with a heart'. Such a choice comes from knowing your needs and recognizing which are an expression of the inner self and which are merely a by-product of your contact with the physical world.

Chapter 6
Beliefs

Beliefs are thoughts that we repeatedly use in interpreting or understanding ourselves and our experiences. They are statements that we make to ourselves about our reality. They could also be thought of as assumptions or expectations. We use beliefs to predict future events, as well as to explain what has happened in the past. They are the guide posts for much of our behavior. For this reason, beliefs form an important part of our mental structure. By taking the same event and viewing it from the context of different beliefs, we can create completely different realities. It may be difficult to comprehend the extent to which our entire reality is built on a web of beliefs. It is important to examine this closely, especially in this age of media, artificial intelligence, and conspiracy theories.

To illustrate this, let us consider the example of an individual who believes that by working hard, he will be able to gain all the things that will bring happiness. This belief will exert a powerful influence on his behavior. It will direct his energy in ways that are dictated by his beliefs. He will overlook other possible ways of achieving happiness. It will lead him to look outside himself for happiness—to see happiness as a gift bestowed externally. Thus, striving to earn and to own objects will become very important. Power may become important as a means to have more.

Compare this with a person who believes that he might achieve happiness through relationships with other people. To this person, what is important is whatever enhances his relationships with others. Having things will be of secondary importance to being with people. Sharing will be of greater importance than owning. Power may not be important or might be important for different reasons. It might be used as a way of protecting the self against loss of esteem or loss of relationships.

Each of these two people is experiencing very different realities. Even if they were to go through exactly the same events, they would experience the events differently.

Beliefs are the mechanism by which we structure reality, both personally and in groups. Our physical perceptions are like a Rorschach inkblot which is given meaning by our way of thinking about it. We are free to exercise our creativity in our way of thinking about reality. There is no absolute truth in any of the interpretations given to our perceptions. Each person interprets reality in unique ways. This diversity is to be encouraged, for it is a reflection of the creativity of each individual. All knowledge is ultimately personal.

In order to fully appreciate the way in which beliefs form our individual reality, it is helpful to discuss them in two separate categories. The first category is personal beliefs while the second is group or mass beliefs.

Personal Beliefs

In discussing personal beliefs, an attempt will be made to consider the individual as though he were uninfluenced by his social environment, at the same time recognizing that this is an impossible task. It will also be useful to discriminate between conscious and subconscious aspects of beliefs.

Fully conscious beliefs are within subjective awareness, are able to be examined rationally, and can be displaced by alternative beliefs. They guide behavior but are accompanied by a feeling of being free to choose courses of action.

Fully subconscious beliefs are outside of subjective awareness, are not subject to rational scrutiny, and guide behavior in a fixed and rigid fashion. They are beliefs that are deeply embedded and are generally based on childhood learning. They form much of what we perceive our reality to be.

Every personal belief contains both conscious and subconscious elements. The diagram below illustrates beliefs on a continuum of subconscious through conscious with three different types of beliefs being represented.

Conscious

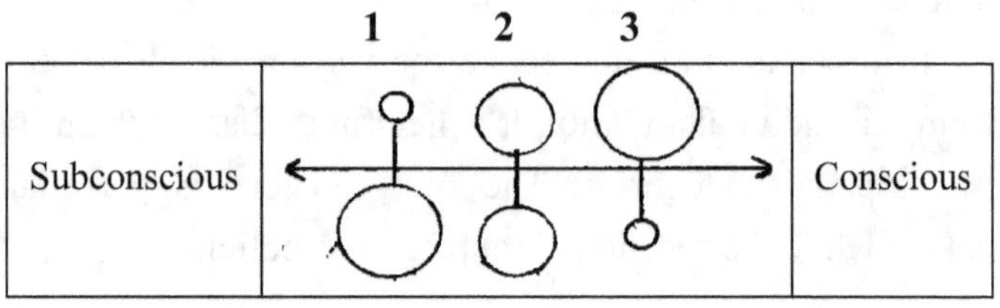

Belief number one has a small conscious element and a large subconscious element so that it would influence behavior in a rigid way and would be free from rational examination. Behavior growing out of this belief would be automatic and inflexible. There are many examples of such beliefs. The attitudes that people hold about themselves are frequently beliefs of this type.

Upon entry into life, the inner self finds itself immersed in a set of circumstances that will be viewed in the light of the needs of this reality, such as the need for love, security, self-esteem, affiliation, meaning, and so forth. These circumstances include such factors as the personalities of our parents and siblings, the community and society that we live in, and the opportunities that will be available to us. They will, in many ways, define the types of experiences we will have. Such factors may remain constant throughout our lives but we will have the opportunity to experience them differently as we focus on different needs.

The beliefs that we hold about ourselves and our experiences are shaped by these circumstances. As a child, each of us was taught certain ways of thinking about ourselves and the world around us. We came to think of ourselves as having certain attributes, talents, and shortcomings. We might come to think of ourselves as being shy, generous, or handsome; as having a musical talent, a gentle disposition, or a bad temper; as being dumb, funny, or ugly. There are many, many such concepts which we might apply to ourselves. We come to believe that some things are possible and some are not. We are provided with a way of looking at the world around us and what limitations we are to expect.

Throughout our lives, these beliefs are adjusted and attuned to our experiences. An obvious example of this on a societal scale is the changes in beliefs that accompany new scientific discoveries or technical innovations. The discoveries of people like Columbus, Galileo, Einstein, and the Wright Brothers have resulted in changes in the beliefs of their contemporaries as the horizon of experience was broadened. On a personal level, each of us adjusts the limitations of our beliefs when we challenge those beliefs and venture into new areas of experience. The person who has always believed she was shy may find that she can successfully hold a job that requires her to talk to other people. The person who believed that he was short-tempered may find that he is patient, tolerant, and understanding when he is asked to help an elderly neighbor. Such new experiences broaden the scope of the possibilities that we see for ourselves.

However, many of the beliefs that we hold about ourselves are so much a part of our thinking that we cannot see them as being changeable. Such beliefs are the ones which most profoundly affect our lives, in that they place unquestioned limitations on our experience. They are also the ones that we are likely to have the least conscious awareness of because they are so intimately interwoven with our being. These are the types of beliefs that are largely subconscious or outside of our normal conscious awareness. Their effect is to make our behavior automatic in situations that are related to the belief. The person who believes that he is unable to learn mathematics will automatically avoid making any real attempt at solving a mathematical problem that is presented to him. The person who believes that her ideas are not as worthwhile as the ideas of others will not make an effort to communicate her ideas.

Belief number three in the earlier diagram is one that has a large conscious element and a small unconscious element. This is the status of new beliefs that we are just beginning to incorporate into our mental structure. We have a high degree of awareness of the belief, for it can only be maintained through this conscious awareness. As soon as we stop thinking about it, it stops influencing our behavior. There is no automatic element in such a belief.

Anyone who has tried to learn a new skill or to change their ideas or behavior will understand how such a belief operates. It requires constant mental concentration on the belief in order for behavior to be influenced. We have no corresponding experience to support the validity of the new belief. For example, if a shy person were to change his belief that other people will disapprove of him, his starting point is one that includes an automatic response to selectively look for disapproval and an absence of experiences in which he saw others as approving of his ideas or behavior. If he attempts to believe that others will approve of his ideas and behavior, he will have to overcome these barriers. This new belief will have little influence on his experiences unless he maintains a conscious effort to interpret his experiences in the light of it, to look at that side of the cube. Thus, the advantage of this third type of belief is that it is easily changed. Its disadvantage is that it requires a great deal of mental energy to maintain its effect on our experiences.

The second belief in the diagram combines the best of both extremes of the continuum. A large conscious element means that the belief is contained in conscious awareness and can be changed or altered. Such awareness provides flexibility within the mental structure, which is vital for growth to take place.

In the final analysis, all that ever really changes is our understanding. As understanding expands, the actual events of our lives become less and less important. When we fully understand that we are the creators of our perception and that our perception ultimately determines our experience, it becomes apparent that we will receive the experience we need regardless of what events occur. Such understanding can only be gained through the expansion of self-awareness, through the growth of our awareness of our needs, beliefs, and values. A conscious awareness of all of our beliefs is a truly desirable goal.

The second belief also possesses a large subconscious element that provides stability and energy to the belief, so that it can guide behavior without requiring conscious concentration. This is desirable, provided that there is the conscious recognition that a choice is available, that beliefs are only avenues to experience and we are free to take the path we choose. This second type of belief is the one that most effectively serves the person who holds it. It allows us to enter the circus tent of experiences that the belief will produce, knowing that we can leave when we choose and enter a new tent.

You will note that this optimum state can be arrived at from two different directions. It can be reached by increasing awareness of beliefs of the first type that are already providing automatic direction to our experiences. It can also be reached by allowing new beliefs to become more firmly established in the subconscious. Later in this chapter exercises will be presented to accomplish both of these tasks.

Our growth and development in this reality is a process of growing through various beliefs and needs as our understanding expands. When beliefs are held rigidly, they direct our experience in the same paths over and over again. Strongly held beliefs serve to direct our behavior and influence our perception of events in such a way as to confirm our original beliefs.

For example, a shy person who believes that he is unworthy of receiving praise and attention from others will avoid situations that would make it possible to experience these things. Or someone who is suspicious and distrustful of others because he sees evil in them will experience the evil he sees. Remember, beliefs are the constructs by which we grant meaning to our experience. Once meaning is created, it will continue to be applied to events and will act as a guide for experience. If you give some thought to how this applies to you, you will appreciate the pervasiveness and power of this process.

If we can be open in examining ourselves, we can begin to identify beliefs that we may wish to change. Each of us has beliefs that produce emotional pain for us. We have areas in which our beliefs lead us to feel that we are being deprived in some way or that we are somehow less worthy or less important than others. We have beliefs that place limitations on our experience, closing off certain avenues to us. There are beliefs that lead us to fear certain possibilities, especially that of our physical death. There are beliefs that lead us to feel that others have power over us or that we are the victims of our life circumstances.

An open-minded attitude that allows all beliefs to be challenged will permit the perception of new possibilities. Such perception will allow more positive or constructive beliefs to be developed. These beliefs should open up new areas of experience. They will not necessarily require that new events take place, although this is certainly possible and likely. More importantly, they will allow for a new perception of events. A new meaning will be granted to events.

But further, one may continue to grow through these positive beliefs until a state of mind is reached wherein one believes all things and yet believes nothing. All beliefs can be seen as temporary, artificial constructs that merely reflect the viewer's perspective. The formulation of beliefs and the meaning they ascribe to reality is like building a boat with which to sail upon the sea of life. Once constructed, we set sail in our little boats, enjoying the security of our handiwork. When we are struck by storms and our boats are sunk, we swim to shore and build a new boat that we hope is bigger and stronger. The process is repeated again and the boat is rebuilt until we recognize that our real security lies in the fact that we know how to build boats.

But, do not be in a hurry to take short cuts to enlightenment. The beliefs that you hold reflect needs that must be resolved before the beliefs can truly change. It is not truly possible, for example, to let go of limiting beliefs before the need for self-acceptance is fulfilled. If one acknowledges and accepts one's needs and beliefs, it is possible to begin working through them by questioning them and ensuring that important needs are met.

Strongly held beliefs exert such a profound effect on our behavior that it is difficult to get a perspective that will allow us to see those effects. When a belief is deeply held, we cannot see how things could be any other way. The hypnotic subject in a deep trance may so strongly believe the hypnotist's suggestion that he has been burned that he will actually develop blisters.

We can see from this that strongly held beliefs affect even individual cells. Our beliefs deeply condition our entire body to expect certain conditions. The implications of this in the field of health are only now beginning to be realized. The connection between mind and body is intimate. It has long been known that physical responses are associated with emotions and that under prolonged emotional stress; the body may begin to break down. Ulcers, migraine headaches, eczema, and high blood pressure are some well-known examples of the body's response to such emotional stress.

However, more and more examples are surfacing of instances where the course of a disease is interrupted by an alteration or manipulation of a person's beliefs. The most obvious and common example is the use of placebo drugs. Doctors have long known that the mere fact that a patient believes he is receiving treatment for an illness may speed his recovery, even if all he is receiving is a sugar pill.

In the course of our involvement in society around us, we have adopted a number of important beliefs about our health. For example, we know that colds are caused by viruses. We know that colds are contagious. When exposed to someone who has a cold, we expect to catch it also. If we do catch it, we expect to be sick for about three days. We will need medicines to relieve our symptoms. Subconsciously, we may welcome the cold if it means that we can escape from a dreary job for a few days. All of these factors contribute to preparing the body to be ill.

In general, we have turned over control of our health to the medical profession. We have come to believe that our health is a delicate state which requires considerable assistance to maintain. And yet, most doctors realize that their medical interventions only assist the healing process, that healing is a natural bodily function. It is a function that is very closely connected to the mental state of the individual. Beliefs create a climate of self-fulfilling expectations wherein their suggestive quality leads to the expected outcome.

Scientific knowledge has most certainly made important contributions to our way of life, but it has, in some instances, brought with it a heavy determinism that closes off certain possibilities because we see them as impossible. There are many examples of spontaneous remissions of diseases that are medically inexplicable. Our beliefs form an important part of the mental fabric to which our body responds.

An important step in changing our reality is to become aware of the beliefs we hold regarding it. Listed below are some general categories within which each of us holds a variety of beliefs. Try to identify at least one belief that you hold in each of these areas. Write them down. Concentrate especially on the areas which are of concern to you. Be as open and honest with yourself as you can be.

Remember, the most important beliefs to become aware of are the ones that are mostly subconscious. These will be the ones that will be most difficult to identify. For this reason, the best way to do this exercise is to take your time and think about it for several days, writing down ideas as they come to mind. A few minutes of meditation each day is a useful way to expand self-awareness. Any opportunities that you have to discuss your feelings and beliefs with a trusted friend or family member can be helpful in clarifying your thoughts. Another person can often point out beliefs that we have not recognized.

Interaction with others:

Examples: I believe that others will disapprove of my thoughts and feelings.

I believe that others must always approve of me in order for my needs to be met.

Personal qualities:

Examples: I believe that angry outbursts are a natural part of my behavior.

I believe that my physical appearance is not pleasing to others.

Health:

Examples: I believe that I catch every contagious disease that goes around.

I believe that my health problems will be very much like those of my parents.

Work:

Examples: I believe that the worth of my job is measured by the amount of money I am paid and the social status associated with it.

I believe that there are parts of my job that are hard for me to cope with.

Family life:

Examples: I believe that my spouse does not understand some of my thoughts and feelings.

I believe that it is necessary for me to make most of the decisions in my family.

The past:

Examples: I believe that my parents did not provide the kind of love I needed.

I believe that my failures in various areas show that I do not have the capabilities required in those areas.

The future:

Examples: I believe that the future is likely to bring some type of hardship.

I believe that happiness lies somewhere in the future with the improvement of present circumstances.

In the exercise that you have just done, you have, hopefully, become aware of some of your beliefs. While it is unlikely that you have learned anything startling about yourself, you should recognize that these are ways in which you have chosen to think about your reality. They are not absolutes. They are merely one way to interpret your experience.

Are there, among these beliefs, any that you would like to change? Are there any new beliefs that you would like to establish in your mental structure? Choose one to begin working on. Rewrite it in a way that will allow you to see your experience in a new light, to allow you more personal freedom.

Examples:

I believe that others will disapprove of me becomes I believe that it is most important that I understand and accept my thoughts and feelings.

I believe that angry outbursts are a natural part of my behavior becomes I can come to understand what triggers my anger and I have a choice as to how I express my anger.

I believe that the worth of my job is measured by the amount of money I am paid and the social status associated with it becomes I believe that the importance of my job is determined by the kinds of experiences it offers me and what I do with those experiences.

I believe that my spouse does not understand some of my thoughts and feelings becomes I believe that I can make myself understood by my spouse.

I believe that the future is likely to bring some type of hardship becomes I believe that I can cope with and benefit from whatever the self-awareness future brings.

When you have rewritten the belief, spend between five and fifteen minutes focusing your attention completely on the new belief. Repeat it a few times to yourself. Review your past experiences in order to seek out experiences that would support the new belief. Use those experiences to make that new belief feel true. Visualize yourself as you would be if you accepted that belief. Imagine yourself being the person who believes that. Focus on the feelings it brings. Let that belief be a part of you for this brief time. Continue examining past events in the light of that new belief in order to see how they could substantiate it. Allow this belief to form a new gestalt on past events. When you are finished, do not think further about it. Set the matter aside but repeat the exercise once or twice a day for a week.

Group Beliefs

The function of beliefs is not one which is restricted to individuals. Beliefs also play an important role in the creation of a consensus reality that serves as a backdrop to the personal reality of each individual. Consensus reality consists of the beliefs that are most commonly held about ourselves and the world around us. For example, the belief that life is a precious gift, that should be saved at all costs, is one that is widely held in Western society. Hospitals, advanced medical technology, highly trained physicians, emergency medical services, and laws protecting human life are some of the outgrowths of this belief. These phenomena form a part of the native environment in which you are formulating your definition of self.

On the more destructive end of the continuum, there are group beliefs that support racist attitudes and behavior. This is powerfully communicated in the book *Rising out of Hatred: The Awakening of a Former White Nationalist* by Eli Saslow. It is well worth reading to understand how a group context maintains beliefs and how difficult it is to change this.

As a participant in a group or society, it is often difficult to see that such beliefs are not absolute. They are merely one way of perceiving reality, one way of organizing our experience. Returning to the previous example, we know that beliefs are not universally shared. The Inuit people traditionally required that people who become too old to care for themselves must take their own lives. If they could not, then it was the duty of a relative to assist them. The Japanese have held honor to be more important than life. Consider how many wars have been fought over religious beliefs. Our ethnocentrism often leaves us blind to the fact that there are many equally valid beliefs that may describe the same phenomenon.

When a belief is widely shared by the members of a group or society, a web of energy is formed that has a powerful influence on the personal reality of each member of the group. Beliefs do possess energy. If energy is defined, as it often is, as the capacity to do work, one only needs to look at what a belief produces to see that they do, indeed, possess energy.

Earlier, it was pointed out that the belief in the value of life has produced a number of lifesaving and life-protecting institutions and procedures in our society. The belief that certain kinds of knowledge are important for all people to have has produced the institution of schools and the institutional enforcement of compulsory education. The institutions of society are a reflection of the mass beliefs of the individuals who live in the society. When these beliefs are coherent throughout society, there is less social unrest.

The energy web of a group belief is formed by the creation of bonds of agreement between the members of the group. These bonds of agreement form a web between people that directs their actions in a common fashion. In the language of physics, they express their energy by deceasing the entropy of the system. Each member of a group participates in an energy network that both directs the activity of the group and sustains the belief of each member of the group. Jointly, they create a reality that coincides with the nature of the belief. The energy network for a single belief is illustrated in the accompanying diagram.

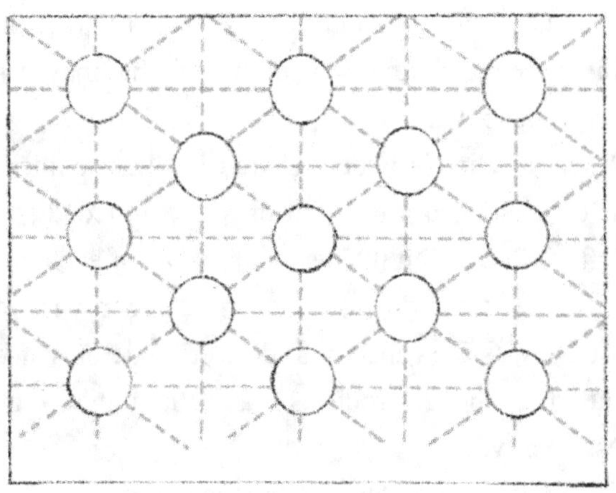

Consider each circle in the diagram to be a separate person and the dotted lines connecting the circles to be bonds of agreement between these individuals about the particular belief. When a belief is energized by a complete network of agreement, such as in the diagram, it exerts a powerful influence on the perception and behavior of the group members. For example, the belief that it is necessary for children to receive an education would be energized by many bonds of agreement.

Look at the diagram for a few minutes and try to visualize a mass belief such as this as an energy system. Consider each bond of agreement as containing energy. The bonds of agreement about the belief form a web of energy that exerts a powerful influence on our behavior. It becomes very difficult not to act in accordance with the belief. There are an infinite number of beliefs and the energy systems for these beliefs are overlaid on each other.

Individuals may or may not participate in the energy system for each belief. The systems of agreement with various beliefs that we, as individuals, participate in are, to some extent, what attracts us to other people. We are drawn to people who agree with us.

In order to explore these ideas further, let us look at two different levels at which this phenomenon is expressed. The first is within families and the second is at a societal level.

Family

Each family possesses a unique set of beliefs that are shared by the family's members. These beliefs are about the family's history and the nature of the individuals in the family. They also describe the kind of interaction that is desirable within the family and the family's interaction with the society that surrounds it. These familial beliefs are an important factor in the formation of the mental structure of each family member.

I would like to describe a dream that I feel says some important things about the way in which we relate to each other. It is particularly relevant to relationships within families.

I dreamed of two ladies dancing in relationship to each other without touching. They each held a mirror in one hand which was always positioned so that they saw themselves instead of the other person. They wished to have sexual contact with each other but were confronted with the obvious problem that they were both of the same sex. The problem was solved when realizing that the other person was seen as a reflection of themselves, they recognized that the other person could be made into whatever they wanted them to be.

This dream has special significance for me because of the powerful message that I feel it expresses. I do not feel that the sexual aspect of the dream has any real importance. The real meaning of the dream lies in what it says about human interaction. We dance life's dance, never really touching each other. When we look at others, we see ourselves. We project onto others our needs, fears, and beliefs and make them into whatever we want them to be. The people who surround us are tools that we use in the externalization of our internal reality. We see them in the way we need to see them.

Nowhere is this more apparent than in the close emotional relationships that exist in families. I will try to illustrate this with some examples.

Annette had been raised in a family where the central character was a domineering, controlling, and emotionally abusive father. Although she struggled against his treatment of her, she did come to adopt his belief that she was not a worthwhile person and needed someone to tell her what to do. Her involvement with Eric at sixteen years of age became a vehicle by which she could escape from her father. At the same time, however, her need to be loved by her father meant that some of the qualities that attracted her to Eric were very similar to her father.

Eric had been raised in a family that provided little emotional support. He was criticized severely by his parents but was free to dominate his younger brothers and sisters. He came to believe that his personal worth depended upon the extent to which others would support his goals and methods. He believed that their failure to do so was an insult to his self-esteem. Eric and Annette's beliefs about themselves fit together like a hand in a glove. Annette's belief that she needed someone to tell her what to do led to her acceptance of Eric's belief system. Her underlying need to win her father's love and approval kept her struggling to find ways to please Eric. On the occasions when she would disagree, Eric would become more and more abusive until her agreement was achieved. His belief system required that it be so.

When Eric and Annette had children, the children also became part of the familial belief system. Their observation of the interaction between Eric and Annette, as well as their own experiences, reinforced the same beliefs. The addition of the children to the family strengthened the beliefs by increasing the number of bonds of agreement. The children came to share the belief with Annette that Eric was a tyrant who must be placated. They also shared Eric's belief that Annette's opinions need not be heeded. Underneath these beliefs, they also shared both Eric and Annette's belief that neither parent was a person who was worthy of respect.

Each family shares a number of beliefs about the individuals who are a part of it. One family member may be believed to be shy, another intelligent, another artistic, another bad-tempered, and so forth. These beliefs often become part of a self-perpetuating system, especially if that belief is shared by the person to whom it is directed. For example, when our daughters were young, one tended to not talk much around other people while her sister showed an unrestrained enthusiasm for conversation. The natural response would have been to believe that one child was shy while the other was outgoing. Such a belief would have solidified the pattern of behavior, making it much more difficult to change. The outgoing daughter was already pleased to do all the talking for her younger sister. To have defined the younger one as shy would have imparted resistance to change to the behavior. It would have suggested a deficit in her character that she needed to be protected against. It would have ignored the underlying reasons for the behavior. An alternative way to handle the behavior would be to say, "No, she is not shy. She just chooses not to talk now."

Any qualitative description of another person suggests a belief about the nature of that person. When that description is shared by family members, an expectation is created that can be self-fulfilling. If a person is believed to be bad-tempered, he is given permission to lose control of himself. He is also deprived of opportunities to learn to control his temper because others avoid discussing anything with him that they fear may anger him. From my experience, it seems that wherever one extreme exists, its opposite is not far away. Any extreme trait in one person is likely to be meeting the needs of another person close by. The angry tyrant highlights the existence of the understanding saint. The introvert and the extrovert meet each other's needs, especially when the extrovert speaks for the introvert.

When one person attempts to change their behavior in the context of a family, the beliefs that the other family members hold can present a major obstacle to change. On the other hand, an alteration in familial beliefs can open new doors to its members. If the family members can see the best in one another, those positive qualities can come to be expressed. An understanding of one's own needs allows others the space to grow in the ways that they need to.

Familial beliefs also define the manner in which communication takes place and the way feelings are expressed. Some families share the belief that anger must not be openly expressed. Others require that love or sadness be covered up. Children must not question their parent's decisions. Disagreements between parents should not be discussed in front of children.

There are many such beliefs that govern the activity of a family. The more such beliefs that the members of a family share, the more structured or rigid the interaction of the family members will be. These beliefs require that individuals behave in certain ways, which often puts unnecessary restrictions on their modes of expression. They may even require that individuals in the family not be aware of certain feelings.

Consider the following example. Sonya had been abandoned by her husband when her four children were all under ten. She received no support from him and found it impossible to live on her welfare allowance. Having no real job skills, she earned a minimal wage at her job. The family could afford only the bare essentials. They lived on the upper floor of a house and Sonya slept in a windowless attic. It was necessary to ride a bus to work. The bus trip was an hour each way.

Sonya became desperately depressed. She frequently contemplated taking her life. It was only the responsibility she felt for her children that kept her alive. Her three daughters recognized her desperate state of mind and a belief was born into the family. It was that every possible step must be taken to avoid upsetting Sonya. This belief was shared by Sonya as well as the three girls. The girls became model children. They were almost totally self-reliant and never expressed any feelings of sadness or anger in front of their mother. However, they paid a heavy price for their adherence to the belief. There was no one to provide any emotional support to them in dealing with their own problems. It was necessary to hide any strong feelings that they had.

The only one who did not share this belief was Sonya's son, who seemed to make constant emotional demands upon her. He became the focus of all the problems that the family experienced. His disruptive behavior was seen as being responsible for his mother's depression. His sisters were angered by his behavior because it violated their beliefs. They soon came to share the belief that his actions were the cause of the unhappiness that everyone in the family felt. They placed tremendous pressure on him to stop upsetting their mother.

In this example, the communication of feelings is clearly governed by the beliefs that are shared by most of the family members. A reality is created in which one member of the family is seen as needing protection. The one person who does not conform to this reality is pressured to accept the belief and to act in accordance with it.

Every family has its own set of beliefs about its members and about communication and roles within the family. Becoming aware of these beliefs and seeing them as changeable can create newfound freedom for oneself as well as for other family members. Whenever we attribute traits to other people, we create an atmosphere of limitation. Even positive traits can create such limitations. It can be burdensome to be part of a group belief that sees you as gentle, understanding, or kind. It may require that you suppress all natural experiences of anger, annoyance, and confusion. True freedom requires that all such beliefs be seen as temporary constructs that are completely changeable. When this is accomplished, you liberate not only yourself but those around you as well. When beliefs about patterns of communication are recognized as such, new possibilities of expression are created. The number of conscious choices that you have available to you is broadened.

The questions that follow are suggested as a vehicle to expanding your awareness of the group beliefs that exist in your own family. They may be applied to your present family structure as well as to your family of origin. Applying them to your family of origin may help you become aware of limiting beliefs that you continue to apply to yourself. It would be most helpful to write the answers down.

1. What are the notable qualities or characteristics that your family as a group, identifies about each of its members?
2. What expectations are created for each individual by these descriptions?
3. Do any of the qualities of two people serve the needs of each other?
4. Have you ever observed any exceptions in the behavior of any of the individuals to the qualities which have been ascribed to them?
5. To what extent do these group beliefs meet your own needs?
6. What beliefs does your family hold about the expression of anger, sadness, and love?
7. What limitations do you personally feel about the expression of feelings in your family?
8. What limitations do others experience about the expression of feelings?
9. How would you describe the personal reality of each other member of your family?

Society

Group beliefs provide the foundation for any cooperative action in society. They coordinate the activities of the individuals within a family, group, community, country, and even groups of countries, allowing for the creation of influences that affect all the members of that grouping. Social institutions such as schools, hospitals, and the courts are an outgrowth of group beliefs. Even systems of government are based upon fundamental concepts that are widely shared.

In some areas, these beliefs are constantly shifting and changing as more or less people support them, as new competing beliefs come and go. In other spheres, certain basic beliefs are firmly established and are subscribed to by nearly all the members of that group. Examples of this latter type of belief in Western society would include such concepts as freedom of speech, the idea that all members of society should be provided with equal opportunity, and the belief that each person should have an equal voice in the governmental process.

When there are many bonds of agreement energizing a particular belief, it is able to direct the activities of its adherents in such a way as to create a reality that corresponds to it. For example, the belief that objective knowledge is not only valuable but necessary, to achieve a quality of lifestyle is widely shared in modern industrialized society. It has resulted in the creation of educational institutions to provide for mandatory education, as well as universities and colleges that are readily accessible to the general population. Energy is directed from each person who accepts this belief toward creating and utilizing opportunities for education. At the same time, this energy has also contributed toward creating a society wherein the need for education is a reality. Education has come to be used as a prerequisite to employment. Financial remuneration and education have become closely linked. The belief is a two-edged sword that has created the reality that it describes.

This is not to suggest that the belief should, therefore, be changed. We may continue to choose this as the reality that we wish to experience. It is, however, important to retain the recognition that this is only one way of describing reality. This is only one of an infinite number of realities that may be created by means of our shared beliefs. Every shared belief contributes toward creating an aspect of what we see as 'objective' reality just as our personal beliefs serve to create our personal reality. Society and its institutions are a reflection of its members. Their nature is a reflection of the beliefs that are most widely shared. Because of the energy that they direct, widely shared beliefs have a powerful influence in shaping the reality that we experience. Our entire societal way of life is directed by the beliefs that we share.

But there are also competing beliefs that create conflict within and between societies. Historically, there have been competing belief systems between religions that have been the source of wars. There are competing belief systems in economic theory that have led to conflicts between left-wing and right-wing elements. This led to the Cold War which dominated world events for decades after World War II and that continues to be a source of conflict in modern times.

On a smaller scale, there are competing personal belief systems on issues like vaccination, gun control, immigration, climate change, crime, poverty, and conspiracy theories with groups of people on each side of the issue holding adamant views. The perspectives involved in these issues are supported by selective attention to information that supports the issue in question and ignoring competing information.

However, there are still many areas where we remain passive creators of a reality that we wish were different. Within the web of a group belief, each individual has equal power to instigate change. Quiet complicity in the face of a belief that we do not want to support is the same as giving tacit agreement. Leaders are people who are able to utilize group beliefs to support their aims and objectives. An effective leader is someone who is able to spin a web of belief that most of the members of the group will support because it appeals to the needs of each individual who supports it.

Appealing to our need to see good and bad are a series of beliefs that pit us, the 'good guys', against them, the 'bad guys'. This illusion is being used to justify enormous destructive capabilities, just as it has been used through the centuries to enlist combatants for a multitude of egocentric causes. This can only change if we stop seeing the world in black and white and examine issues from a variety of different perspectives. The challenge in debating competitions has always been to be able to look at an issue from two or more different sides. Societal change can come about only as a result of a change in consciousness on the part of its individual members. There is no other way. Each of us, individually, is as much a creator of society as we are victims of it. Every time we share agreement, whether overtly or covertly, with others on the beliefs that guide our social reality, we reinforce those beliefs and contribute to their energy. We are all equally responsible for the products of those beliefs.

Leaders can only lead those who understand and share their goals and motivations.

The beliefs that we support and participate in are descriptive of who we are as individuals. Society is the collective description of our personal realities. Social change must begin with personal change. When your beliefs change, you can have an important effect on the prevailing group beliefs. Your agreement with these beliefs is an important source of energy for the belief. It is just as important as the agreement of any other individual. Your agreement has served to reinforce the conviction of others in their belief. When you no longer support the belief, you weaken the belief of all those with whom you communicate. This effect has been illustrated in the accompanying diagram.

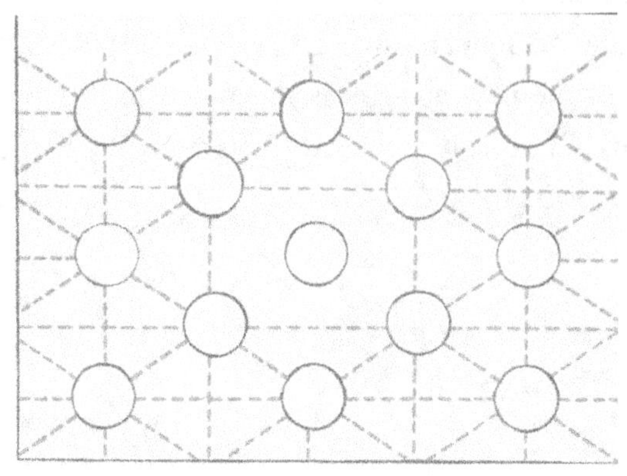

It can be seen that when one person stops agreeing with that idea, he weakens the belief of all those around him. Each of those people now has one less person agreeing with them. The belief loses some of its energy. The next pages illustrate what happens when this person shares his new idea with someone else in the group and wins their support for it.

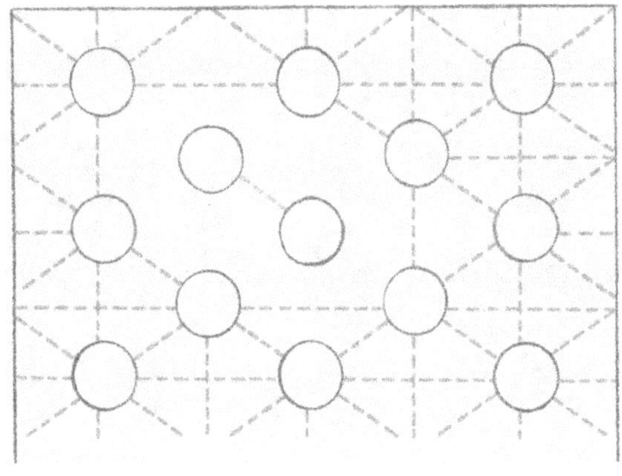

Each successive person who supports the new belief contributes to reducing the energy of the old ideas. The growth of the new concept is illustrated in the remaining diagrams. Eventually, societal structures will be influenced by this growing belief.

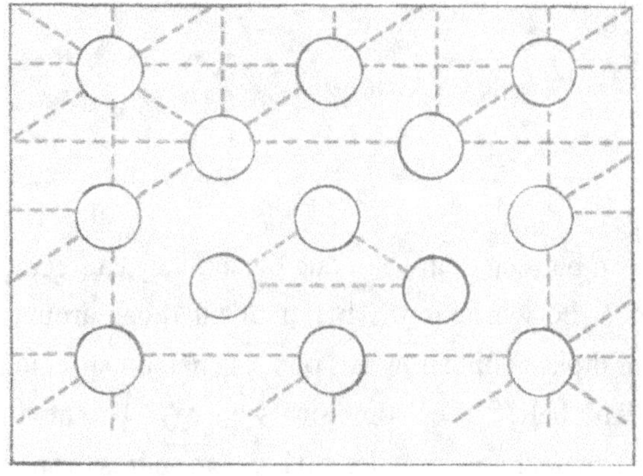

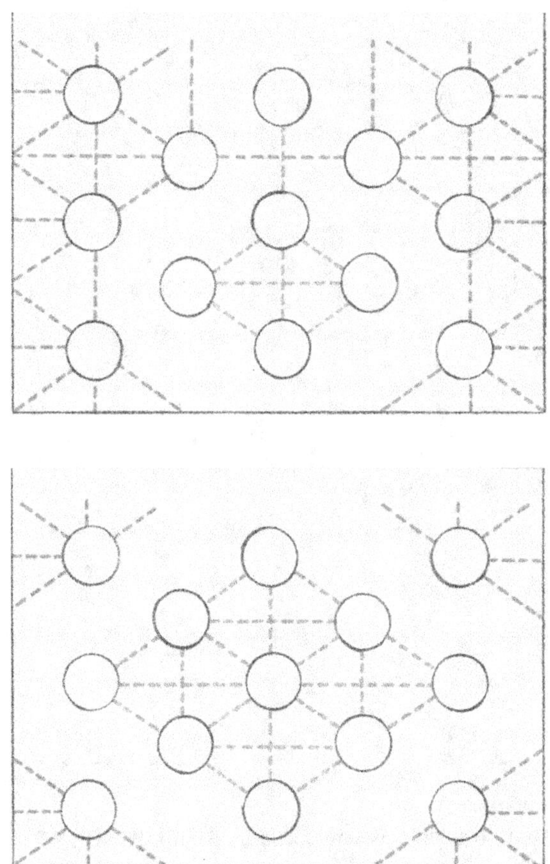

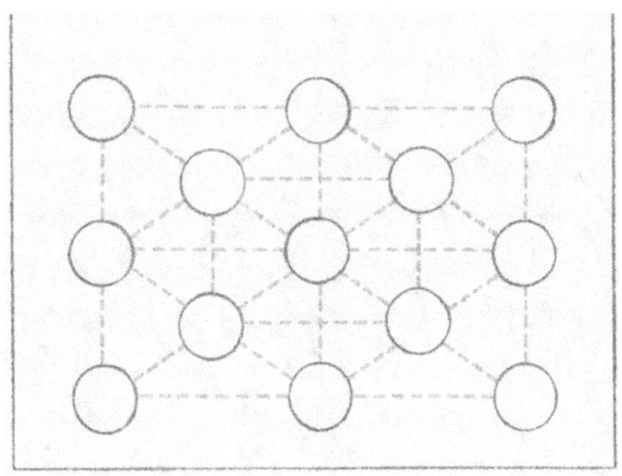

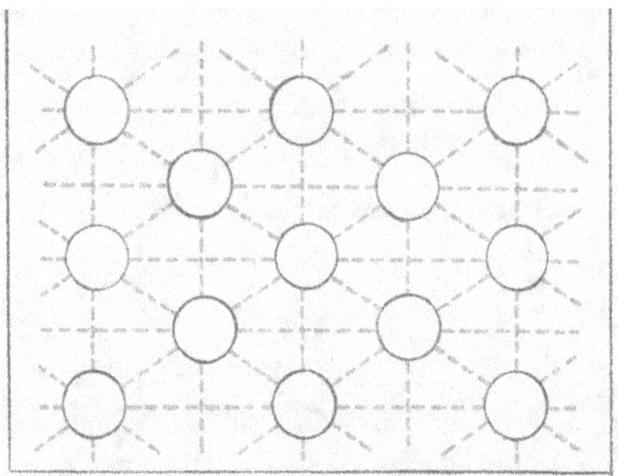

This is the process of change. If an attempt were made to impose societal structures based on the new belief on a group that unanimously agreed on the old ideas, these structures would be rejected. It is only when sufficient agreement is established within a group that the products of that belief will begin to unfold.

As an exercise, take some time to write down some of the group beliefs that contribute to your collective reality.

These may be rather subtle and difficult to identify, especially if you have a strong commitment to them. Be aware of the ways in which you support these beliefs through your agreement with others. Try to see these beliefs as only one possible way of perceiving your experience and look for some alternatives.

Chapter 7
Emotions

I have not yet covered the issue of emotions, which are an important aspect of understanding the human psyche. Before we start, I want to emphasize that the resolutions that I suggest in the following discussion are not intended to be glib or to suggest that one can quickly and easily change emotional reactions. Emotional patterns are persistent and require concentrated effort over a lengthy period of time to change. The resolutions that I suggest are drawn from the field of clinical psychology and have generally been shown to be effective in treating emotional problems.

Emotions arise from the more primitive parts of the human brain and thus, are not under the easy control that cognitive functions are. They are a strongly motivating factor in human behavior and interact with beliefs by stimulating and reinforcing them. When emotions arise, we look for reasons for them and this causes new beliefs to form. At the same time, beliefs can stimulate emotions and emotional arousal reinforces the belief. So let us look at some of the major types of emotion.

Fear/Anxiety

Fear is perhaps the most primary emotion because it has historically had a significant role in the survival of the species, for that matter, all species. The function of fear is to protect an individual from real-life danger. But fears tend to be much broader than that. We form many fears that have nothing to do with survival. Life circumstances have changed with the evolution of society, so there now are relatively few situations where our existence is threatened. There still are some realistic fears in this category, such as the fear of venomous snakes or the fear of heights. But even these can be taken to disabling extremes. The more common fears now are probably those related to social interaction. Fears can also be stimulated by frequent exposure to horror films and negative news. In these days of the internet, there are fears that arise because of exposure to false or misleading information, as is seen in conspiracy theories.

The natural reaction to fear is avoidance. We steer clear of situations and things that cause fear and anxiety. But what is the effect of this? Whenever we avoid something that we fear, we experience negative reinforcement. We have essentially told ourselves that if we had actually encountered the fearful situation or stimulus, something bad or painful would have occurred. When we avoid the situation, we unconsciously tell ourselves that it is a good thing to have done so. This serves as a reinforcement that maintains the fear.

It follows that the best resolution of a fear is to actually encounter the stimulus or situation. But if we encounter the fearful stimulus and are overwhelmed with fear, this also serves to reinforce the fear. The first step in overcoming fear is to learn to regulate one's level of emotional arousal. High arousal has the effect of maintaining anxiety or fear because it triggers patterns of thinking that support the emotional state. Reducing levels of arousal can be accomplished in a number of ways. The easiest way is through breathing exercises.

When you are in a state of fear or anxiety (another form of fear), the sympathetic or involuntary nervous system is activated and it creates a number of bodily changes. Breathing becomes shallow, heart rate increases, digestive changes occur, perspiration increases, muscle tension increases, and so on. We do not have any voluntary control over most of those changes. They happen without any effort on our part and we cannot change most of them, except for muscle tension and the rate of our breathing. So the action of the sympathetic nervous system can be slowed by muscle relaxation or alterations in breathing patterns.

One simple method is to breathe deeply and slowly. This can be accomplished by inhaling deeply and slowly. When the inhale is complete, hold your breath to the count of five and then slowly exhale. Repeat this several times and you should notice that feelings of anxiety are diminished.

As to muscular tension, many years ago, psychologists Wolpe and Lazarus developed a deep muscle relaxation technique to counter this. The exercise consists of tensing and then relaxing different muscle groups in the body. Start with tensing the muscles in your feet and holding the tension until the muscles start to tire before relaxing them. Progress through the body from there, the calves, thighs, stomach, chest (by inhaling and holding the breath), fists, forearms, biceps, neck, jaw, and facial muscles. In each case, the muscular tension needs to be held until the muscles are fatigued before relaxing. Even people who do not have obvious problems with anxiety will find that they hold tension in various muscle groups and can benefit from the exercise.

A third method of learning to let go of tension is meditation. The object of meditation has more to do with learning to regulate the thoughts that lead to anxiety and fear. In meditation, you need to sit comfortably with the back in an upright position. This could be on a meditation cushion or in a chair. Meditation requires a point of focus. This can consist of an object that has no particular significance, such as a rock or a candle. When I first meditated, I used a small brass Buddha incense burner. A mantra (a sound that is repeated) can also be used. When I first meditated, I would inhale deeply and then say OM in a long, slow exhale.

Another point of focus is the breath. Before starting, it is important to set a timer and to make the meditation session at least 15 minutes long. It takes a while to settle the body and mind. You must also vow not to interrupt the meditation session until the time is complete. You will find that your mind does not really want to go through this process and you will start to have thoughts like, "I have better things to do." The meditation begins with breathing deeply and slowly. If you are focusing on your breath, you might imagine inhaling through one nostril and out the other. Keep your focus entirely on your breath or the object you have chosen. Almost immediately you will find that thoughts will intrude. When they do, you remind yourself that you are thinking and you let go of the thoughts, no matter how invasive they are. During meditation, no thought is important. This is what you are training yourself to do, to be able to let go of thoughts without giving them energy. With persistent practice of meditation, you may experience moments of clarity where all you experience is the meditation process without the mental jumble that usually occupies our minds. You will gradually learn to experience the inner self rather than the conscious mind.

These three techniques are useful in training yourself to relax and not be overpowered by fear and anxiety. When you feel that you are able to regulate your emotions, exposure to the feared stimulus or situation is the next step. This needs to be done in a gradual way. For example, if someone is afraid of the water, you would not start by pushing them into the deep end of the pool. You might take them to the beach where they can play in the sand and light surf and they can gradually move into deeper water. Learning coping skills like swimming will also be important.

If, for example, the anxiety relates to social situations, such as occurs in conditions like generalized anxiety disorder or agoraphobia, there should be a graduated introduction to social situations, going from one-to-one meetings with a trusted person to being around two or three familiar people, to being in a non-challenging outdoors event like sitting in a park, to small group events with less familiar people, and so on. The important thing is that the person relaxes as completely as possible in each situation. Again, the objective is to be able to be in each of these situations while regulating anxiety by relaxation or breathing techniques. If anxiety becomes uncontrolled, it is better to exit the situation and use relaxation techniques to calm down rather than to experience panic, which will reinforce the anxiety response.

It is important to recognize thoughts that contribute to anxiety or fear. For example, the socially anxious person might say to them self. 'Everybody thought what I said was stupid' after speaking in a social situation. Thoughts such as these amplify social anxiety. If you have engaged in meditation practice, you will find it easier to dismiss these thoughts rather than putting energy into them.

Many fears and anxieties have little rational basis and are the products of negative patterns of thought. But there are also fears and anxieties that have an actual basis. Individuals who have been through traumatic situations or who have been the victims of abuse can be triggered into anxious states by stimuli that remind them, consciously or unconsciously, of the traumatic situation. This can be particularly difficult if the trauma was experienced early in childhood and the person does not have any conscious memory of it. In cases like this, it is probably best to see a qualified therapist for help, but some relief can be gained by relaxing oneself deeply and then allowing for a mental review of the traumatic situation. Doing so on several occasions can reduce the emotional impact of the trauma. The point is to go from the sequence 'thought > emotional distress > avoidance' to 'thought > emotional distress > calming > thought > emotional distress > calming' with the emotional distress gradually diminishing.

Lastly, there are generalized anxiety reactions that people experience when they think of their existence or of the future. This is known as existential anxiety. Much of this anxiety is generated by focusing one's attention on the future rather than on the present moment. None of us know what the future will be, but if we can stay in the present moment and let the future unfold as it will, much of this anxiety can be alleviated. This will be discussed further in the chapters that follow.

Before moving on, I should point out that there are some physiological-based or drug or alcohol-induced causes of anxiety. If you do not take care of yourself with regard to nutrition, sleep, and rest, you will be more prone to anxiety and fear. There are also some physical disorders that cause anxiety, such as hyperthyroidism. Some of the major mental illnesses (disorders caused by disruptions of the neurotransmitters of the brain), such as schizophrenia, can cause intense feelings of anxiety. Such physiological anxiety disorders are best addressed by medical or psychiatric consultation.

Anger

Anger is perhaps the most destructive emotion. It can evolve into hate and rage. Hatred is something that can be learned as one grows up and is often based on stereotypes and generalizations. This type of hatred does not necessarily involve any actual experience with the object of hatred. Rather, it can be a mental set or cognitive readiness to react to certain stimuli. In other words, hatred is a mental habit. Hatred is reinforced by selective attention to things that reinforce the mental set. For example, a racist person may never come into contact with a person of a particular race but the racist attitude is maintained by selective attention to negative information about the race in question without thought as to whether that information is valid as a general description of all people in that race.

Much of the anger that people experience grows out of frustration. We are trying to achieve certain goals and things that threaten to block our goals become the source of frustration and anger. This may be situational or might be generalized. How you think about the situation determines the level of anger and the likelihood that it will generalize to include a wide range of situations.

For example, when I was younger, I would feel angry toward aggressive drivers who seemed to be in a hurry. Then I thought about times when I have been late and wanted to get somewhere quickly, or about times when there are medical emergencies. I began to look at aggressive drivers as people who feel the need to get somewhere quickly and I found that it was better to let them get on their way without interruption than to feel angry about their actions. I may be wrong about some of those people, but it is more important that I do not let them leave me in a state of anger than it is to try to do something about their aggression.

Sometimes the angry person is not someone who you can easily avoid. They might be a boss, fellow worker, or family member. At some point, you may need to get out of a situation that is filled with another person's anger, but if this is not possible, it is best to try to understand the person and the source of their anger. For example, an angry, abusive parent may have been raised in a family where they were subject to high expectations and abused in the process.

Knowing that this is the only way they know how to parent can help to find ways of not taking their abuse personally and showing them alternatives. Forgiveness is always the best way of dealing with other people's anger and misdeeds, even though this can be a very challenging thing to do.

In dealing with your own anger, it is important to understand the thoughts and expectations that you hold and how this motivates your anger. Individuals who have high standards for themselves or others are the most likely to experience anger. Frustration with not seeing one's expectations met is the seed of anger. Blame serves no useful purpose in dealing with your emotions. It is simply a way of losing your power because blame puts all the responsibility on another person or situation and does not allow for an understanding of how your attitudes and actions have created the emotion.

In terms of dealing with angry and hateful feelings, engaging in the self-regulation procedures described in the previous section is important. Anger also activates the sympathetic nervous system but in a different way than fear. Adrenaline is released into the body and a high level of arousal is created. In order to deal with anger effectively, it is necessary to be able to reduce your level of emotionalism. It is also necessary to recognize and let go of patterns of thinking that contribute to it. Let go of blame and focus on understanding and forgiveness. This will help you to let go of the burden of anger and hatred.

Sadness/Depression

Sadness and depression can have many causes, but a primary one is loss. The most primary sadness is grief. When we lose someone or something that was important to us, we react with grief and this is a normal thing. Sometimes, however, we cannot let go of the grief and we have trouble seeing our lives progressing without the person, thing, or situation. Instead of grief being a periodic mourning, it becomes an ongoing attitude. One of the things that can serve to maintain grief is guilt.

Grief involves a focus on the past. Attention is given to how much better life was prior to the loss. It also involves a pessimistic attitude about the future. As will be discussed in the chapters that follow, the best resolution for grief is to learn to focus on the here and now, the present moment. This is best achieved through meditation or practices such as yoga and tai chi, but one can also just focus on what is happening now. "How does the food I am eating taste?" How does my body feel when I move in certain ways? How does it feel to have the sun shine on me? What are the ambient noises around me? What aromas are in the air?

One form of meditation is walking meditation. This involves walking slowly with your hands folded in front of you and attending to the feeling of your body as you take each step. Again, the object is to let go of thoughts that break your concentration and take you out of the present moment.

Nothing that we can do can change the past and we must learn to move on. It is not disloyal to someone who has passed to let the grief we feel at their passing gradually diminish. If you have lost someone close to you, it will be necessary to readjust your life in many ways and you must allow the transition to take place.

Sadness can be about what we do not have in our lives. Perhaps it is something material or it could be unhappiness with the situation that we find ourselves in. Where sadness transforms into depression is when feelings of guilt and hopelessness develop. If a person does not feel capable of directing their life toward an acceptable future, they despair. Guilt is a critical factor in the transformation from sadness to depression because a focus on guilt involves an expectation that things cannot be undone and the future cannot be better. When I was young, we had an altercation with another group of boys. They were strangers to us and I was scared. We started to throw rocks at them to keep them away. One of the rocks I threw hit one of the boys in the neck and cut him. We ran away as fast as we could. For years afterward, I felt very guilty whenever I thought about the incident. It was many years later before I finally told someone what had happened. I was tearful and overcome with emotion, but after I had done so, the memory no longer had the same emotional power over me. Perhaps this is what is useful about the Catholic tradition of confession.

Psychological research has focused on the concept of learned helplessness. Individuals who do not feel capable of directing their lives are more vulnerable to depression. Learned helplessness can occur because an individual has been raised in an abusive or neglectful manner and they have learned that there is nothing they can do to make their situation better. Being the victim of persistent bullying can have the same effect, particularly if the person is socially isolated.

Learned helplessness can, however, also occur in situations where a child has been indulged and overprotected and has never learned to deal with frustration and to do things for themselves. This can be the long-term effect of preventing children from experiencing disappointment or failure and learning from the experience.

The resolution of depression must involve the development of some new skills, such as assertiveness and general communication abilities. Psychological research has shown that cognitive/behavioral training is at least as effective as antidepressant medication in treating depression. Cognitive/behavioral therapy focuses on the thought patterns and behaviors that induce and support depression. On the cognitive side, negative and self-deprecating thought patterns need to be altered to ways of thinking that offer a more positive and optimistic outlook. On the behavioral side, behavior patterns that accompany depression, such as poor nutrition, social avoidance, inadequate sleep, and lack of exercise, are addressed.

Antidepressant medication has become a common medical way of treating depression. The problem with antidepressant medication as a sole treatment is that it does not involve any skills training, so the mental and emotional patterns that underlie depression are not changed, although alleviation of the emotional distress can give a person the energy to make those changes. Consequently, the best form of treatment for depression involves a combination of medication and cognitive/behavioral training.

Love/loneliness

Love is the emotion that is widely sought, but how people define love varies. Very often, people want the type of love that might be defined as romantic attachment. This is understandable as finding a mate can be thought of as a developmental task. But romantic attachment involves a wide range of motives. It can involve a desire to overcome low self-esteem by having someone love you. It can be confused with sexual motives. It can be a way of resolving dependency needs or fulfilling a need arising from a childhood devoid of nurturing parenting. It can be a matter of enhancing self-esteem through an attachment to a person who is good-looking, popular, or of higher status. It can be a matter of wanting to have someone to dominate and to do one's bidding.

I am not the one to define what love is, but there are some elements to a loving relationship, regardless of the relationship or age differential of the persons involved:

- open communication
- respect for that person and for the decisions that they make in their life
- acceptance of and consideration for their feelings
- encouragement for the person's growth and capacity to learn from their experiences
- trust
- commitment

Achieving a loving relationship involves giving up ego rather than having one's ego enhanced.

Loneliness can be thought of as an emotional/psychic separation from others. It can come from being in an environment where there are no people of a like mind, but it can also occur where people are isolated or where they have cut themselves off from deeper social and emotional involvements. Getting over loneliness often involves making changes to the way that one thinks of and approaches relationships. Individuals with social anxiety often experience loneliness because they are unable to reach out to make connections with others.

The experience of love is something that can be felt through meditation. One might think of our normal busy minds as being like clouds that block the blue sky and the sun. We cannot experience universal love because we are too busy with our ego. As you sit in meditation, there will be moments when the mind is quiet. These are like breaks in the clouds. They might not last very long, but they are a start. With persistent practice in being in the moment and not getting caught up in thought and emotional patterns, the breaks in the clouds can become more extensive. You might even reach a point where you can go for longer periods of time when the only thing that you are experiencing is your inner self in the eternal present moment. Typically, a strong sense of peace and universal love accompanies this experience.

Chapter 8
The Past

In infancy, we hold no particular beliefs about ourselves or the world around us. We are born with the potential to develop in any of a number of different directions. The newborn infant has been likened to a blank slate waiting to be written on or a piece of clay waiting to be molded. This is an oversimplification that denies the inherent talents, abilities, and personality traits that develop in children without any particular coaxing. However, it does convey a sense of the child's dependence upon his environment for his development. Perhaps a more accurate analogy would be to compare a child to a flower bed in which many different kinds of seeds have been sown. Each seed represents a different aspect or potential which may be developed. An aspect will be developed to the extent that it becomes the focal point of the child's consciousness. It will grow in accordance with the amount of attention that is devoted to it.

Our parents take on the responsibility in the early stages of life of helping us to define who we are and, as parents, we become responsible for helping our children define who they are. This does seem to be an interactive process insofar as each individual child seems to bring out different aspects of the parent.

For example, parents often find that they have more patience for one child than another, that they will give one child more freedom and responsibility than another, or that they will protect one child more. This may be associated with the circumstances of the pregnancy and birth, with the quality of the early bonding experience, or with environmental pressures or the child's behavior during infancy. There might be a variety of rational cause and effect explanations, but the fact remains that, as the parent brings out different aspects of the child, so also does the child elicit certain aspects of the parent. It has been my experience in viewing many different families that children seem to challenge their parents in the areas where they most need to grow. A problem child is one in whom his parents see the things about themselves that they are least able to accept. A parent who has difficulty understanding their own anger will not find it easy to accept their child's anger. Anyone who has fears that they have not resolved will tend to culture those same fears in their children.

Parents play a large part in the formation of the mental structure which allows the inner self to interact with the world around it. The way in which this is done is dependent to a large extent on the needs of the parents. Every belief, to some extent, represents a need. The beliefs that each parent shares with his children are based upon his needs to see reality in that way. It is difficult for parents to help their children in areas where they, themselves, have strong needs. For example, a child can be taught self-respect only by parents who respect themselves. If a parent does not respect the worth of his thoughts and feelings, he will teach his children to value the thoughts and feelings of others above his own. Another example is that if a parent has a strong need to be loved, he will have trouble helping his children to feel loved or he may smother them in an attempt to compensate for his own feelings.

Parents share unique aspects of themselves with each separate child, just as children exhibit different qualities with each of their parents. We do not really understand the nature of this interaction. We do not know the extent to which the emphasis should be placed on the parent or the child. It has become apparent to me from seeing numerous families that there is a special relationship between problem children and their individual parents. In most instances, it is one parent in particular who has difficulty with the child. They frequently recognize the irrational nature of their feelings toward the child and may feel tremendous guilt about their behavior in relation to that child. However, when faced with the child they will repeat the same patterns of behavior as if they had no control over their actions. The child elicits feelings within them that they do not understand or know how to cope with.

I have belabored this point somewhat because I feel that it is an important one. All current theories of developmental psychology emphasize a linear cause-and-effect model of events that sees the adult as a product of his past experience. Responsibility for the present is always attributed to past events and circumstances. I would like to explore some alternative ways of looking at this process. This linear cause-and-effect model often seems to result in anger and resentment about past events forcing us into our present circumstances. So let us play a game of imagination and examine some other ideas.

Suppose that time did not really exist in the lineal way in which we experience it. Suppose that all the events of your life existed simultaneously, but that you could create the illusion of cause and effect by the manner in which you focused your attention on various events. This is not necessarily such a far-out idea. Time is merely our experience of sequential change in our environment. If we were completely deprived of all sensory data, our experience of time would become much distorted. People who have been placed in such sensory deprivation environments are able to tolerate only a few hours of it before becoming confused, often experiencing hallucinations. Einstein demonstrated in his theory of relativity that time is relative to the observer and his velocity. Time can be slowed as the observer's velocity increases. In fact, if the observer were to travel at the speed of light, it would be possible to observe what we would think of as an effect before we could observe its cause.

For example, he could watch a bullet hit a target before it was fired from the gun. If you are willing to take such liberties with the construct of time, you could think of your life as being like a lightning bolt that flashes instantaneously across the sky. All the events exist at once, simultaneously. However, you are at liberty to focus on any particular part of the lightning bolt.

If your attention were to be fully focused on one point along the lightning, it would appear that the existence of that point depended upon the pattern that was seen leading up to it. You would then have created the illusion of sequential time, of temporal cause and effect.

Instead of seeing such temporal causative relationships between various events in our lives, it could then be possible to see all events as expressions of needs that are instantaneously spattered throughout our lives like paint flung from a brush. The events of childhood that appear to cause later events are merely an expression of the same need as the later events. Events related to that need will continue to occur until the need is understood and resolved.

Consider the following example. Ruth was the second youngest child of a pioneer family. Born shortly after the turn of the century, her elder brothers had left home by the time she was eight. Times were very tough and her father was frequently away from home trying to earn money to support the family. For some reason, her mother pampered her younger sister while expecting her to take care of the full share of household responsibilities. She deeply resented the preferential treatment that her sister received, especially when she was required to hold a full-time job at age twelve.

Her feelings of bitterness and resentment were further reinforced in her marriage. Ruth married a man who provided her with little emotional or financial support. Her life with him required that she take most of the responsibility for the maintenance of the family. By the time they finally separated, she felt nothing but bitterness toward him. She was desperately poor and was forced to rely on the charity of others to get by. She became very self-conscious about other's opinions of her and believed that people looked down upon her. Friendships were short-lived because of her defensive attitude.

As her children grew up, they avoided contact with her. She lived alone in a small cabin. Her youngest son was the only person whom she felt expressed any love or concern for her. Within a year of his leaving home, he was burned to death in a fire. Her youngest daughter, who also bitterly resented the manner in which she had been raised, had left home indicating that she wanted nothing further to do with her. She was later afflicted with a crippling disease which required intensive care and supervision. Ruth agreed to look after her and they spent the next several years battering each other with their bitterness.

Should we assume, in this example, that there is a temporal causality? It is easy to do so. It appears obvious that each earlier event has contributed to and created the subsequent events.

However, viewing things in that way suggests that her present circumstances can be improved only after all those past events and the feelings they have aroused have been reviewed and rectified. If, instead, we were to view each of these events of Ruth's life as an expression of her needs for love and self-acceptance, it would be possible to focus on those needs that exist right now. It would bring us completely into the present. It would allow for the acceptance of those needs as if they had no history. It would allow Ruth to let go of her bitterness and accept that her reality is based on these unfulfilled needs. As long as the needs are unmet, she will continue to experience reality as if she were unloved as if there are parts of herself that she needs to be ashamed of. Once these needs are met, the events of the past will not have to be different in order for her to experience reality differently. Once these needs are met, she will look at different aspects of events. She will examine a different side of the cube.

If you can accept the game that we have played with time, there can be some real advantages to viewing things in this way. If you can move beyond our customary cause-and-effect reasoning, you can get past seeing yourself as a victim of your past circumstances and training. You are the creator. You have created your perception of those past circumstances, just as you are creating your present perception. If there are similarities between the past and the present, it is because the two are growing out of the same needs and beliefs. It is the needs and beliefs that must change for further perceptions to be different. If there is pain from the past, it is only because the same needs and beliefs continue to be held.

From the focal point of our consciousness, which is the present, the events of the past provide us with the material with which to formulate our definition of ourselves. It is through our interaction with others, as children, that we begin to formulate a conception of ourselves and the world around us. By and large, the child looks to others for beliefs that will help him to understand his experiences. If these beliefs are communicated with flexibility and open-mindedness, the child may develop his own flexibility, which will allow him to see that his experiences can be interpreted in many different ways. If the child's needs are being met through his experiences, he can begin to look at other aspects of each event and to see further learning that can be extracted. The various interpretations that can be placed upon his experiences will allow him different choices as to how to respond. He can begin to learn that he has choices and that he makes choices whether he realizes it or not.

The following paragraph was written by our ten-year-old daughter. I think it illustrates the capacity of children to recognize that events can be perceived in many different ways and that different choices grow out of these different perceptions.

Shopping

I think each person does their own shopping. They pick out a choice and, if they do not like it, they take it back and change it. They pick out habits and, just like food, they eat or get rid of them. You pick out fights and put them back where they belong, just like you put groceries in the cupboard. You pick out feelings and keep them or change them.

The concept of choice is very important in considering the past. Who you are now is a product of the choices that you have made in what you perceive to be the past. All the material that you have at this moment, with which to formulate your definition of self is contained within your past experience. Your choices have directed your perception so as to create a reality that corresponds to your needs. Returning to the example of Ruth, at every point throughout her history, she continued to construct her reality to correspond with her need for love and self-acceptance. At every one of the infinite present moments that are stretched over her life history, she has continued to perceive her experience as though she were not loved and needed to feel criticized. There have been numerous opportunities for her to construe her experiences differently, for her to recognize love, and to feel a sense of self-worth.

However, she has chosen not to seek out these possibilities. Her present reality is such that she continues to view her experiences through these needs. When the needs change, her present reality will change but, further than this, it will open the possibility that the past may change also. When her needs change, she can begin to perceive past events in the light of new needs.

The choices that each of us has made in the past have been based upon the needs that we experienced at that time. Events were selected that corresponded to needs that had current priority. It is useful to consider all the events of your life as products of your own consciousness, as manifestations of your needs and beliefs. If you are willing to consider such a possibility, you can consider all the events of your life as events that you have chosen to experience. Such recognition will enable you to take complete responsibility for your reality. It will allow you to recognize the expression of your needs and beliefs in daily events.

If you are unable to recognize that you have made choices in the past, it will be difficult to see the choices that you are making now.

Frequently, we feel that we have no choice in the events of our lives, that events are forced upon us against our will. We refuse to recognize that we do have alternative choices. We hide from ourselves the fact that our needs and beliefs are involved in the choices we make. One way of developing a greater awareness of the extent to which you have directed the events of your life is to think back to some of the obvious choices you have made, such as choice of job, marriage, or school. Write down what other choices were available to you at that time, even if they seem not to have been reasonable or possible. How did those alternatives conflict with the needs and beliefs that you held then? Do they seem as impossible or undesirable now as they did then? Take each of those alternatives and imagine what your life would have been like if you had followed them. What new beliefs would they have created? What other needs would have been met by these alternatives? What other needs could have been met by the choice you made if you sought alternative perceptions of those events?

Our past experiences have also been important in creating and supporting the beliefs that we hold about reality. Once beliefs have been adopted with any degree of rigidity, they tend to be self-perpetuating through the process of selective perception. We tend to perceive our experiences in such a way as to confirm the beliefs that we already hold. For example, a child who believes that he is loved will perceive discipline as evidence of his parent's concern whereas the child who believes that he is not loved will see it as further evidence of rejection. This process is very important when considering the past. The past exists as a memory bank of experiences that we use to define ourselves. We ignore experiences that would allow us to believe otherwise. The past becomes a reflection of ourselves as we are now. We see it through the needs we presently experience. We use it to support the beliefs we currently hold.

The past exists only through the present and changes as the present changes. In fact, we have many different pasts. The past, as it is viewed through a variety of different needs, feelings, and beliefs, can be seen as many distinct realities. The total experience of any one individual can be used to support many unique perceptions, each of which is a separate reality. Much of our thought is spent living in the past. In particular, we spend a great deal of time reviewing those events and relationships that caused us pain and disappointment and led to the development of negative or limiting beliefs about ourselves. These events and relationships are used to support the present need and to provide justification for the continuation of our negative attitudes.

For example, a person who feels that they were treated unfairly by their parents may continue to recall these events to justify his feelings of pessimism and disappointment in life. Rather than looking at his needs in the present, he focuses on the cause-and-effect relationship which he sees as linking the past with those present experiences. The past appears to justify the present beliefs and the present events revitalize past memories. The interaction continues to stimulate the reality in which feelings of being treated unfairly become a central theme in this person's life. In fact, the reality is based on a need for love and respect. It is this need that links the past and present events. The reality will change only when the need is recognized and resolved. To focus on cause-and-effect relationships between the past and the present is to misdirect your efforts to create change in your reality.

Resolution of the feelings that are attached to events from your personal history can be arrived at by recognizing the needs that were involved in those events. When there is emotional pain attached to events, it is because the same needs continue to exist in the present. It is the needs which must be dealt with. Each of us has experienced relationships and events that have caused us pain and disappointment. On a sheet of paper, write down the name of an individual whose memory causes a strong emotional reaction in you. This may be someone whom you continue to have contact with. It may be a parent, a brother or sister, a lover, a friend, or an enemy. What did you need from this person that you did not receive? Which of your needs were they able to meet? What effect did your experiences with this person have on your beliefs about yourself and upon your reality? What do you believe they needed from you that you were or were not able to provide? What needs do you currently feel that keep you returning to this person or their memory? Close your eyes for a few minutes and ask yourself why you continue to feel this need. Do you wish to continue to hold on to this need? Is it being met in any other way in your life? Are you overlooking the fact that this need has, in fact, been met in other ways? If it has not, could it be met in other ways?

This exercise may be repeated in looking at events that have caused anger, shame, guilt, and fear, but which may not have involved any particular person. Experiences of failure, confrontation, embarrassment, disappointment, ridicule, and so forth which elicit strong emotional reactions can be important points of learning. Such events can highlight aspects of ourselves that we might never have otherwise recognized. Select the event that you would like to examine. Write out a description of the event as you remember it. What needs were you experiencing at the time that the event occurred? How did you interpret the event in relation to those needs? What needs do you feel now in relation to that event? How do these needs continue to stimulate feelings associated with the memory of that event? How can these needs be met now?

You will be prepared to let go of the feelings associated with past relationships and events when you recognize that the needs associated with these memories can be met and are being met in the experiences that you are having each and every moment. If you can let go of these feelings, you will be truly ready to forgive others for their actions in relation to you. You will also be ready to forgive yourself for your behavior in relation to them. It is your willingness to forgive yourself and others that can set you free from any negative bonds that link you to past limitations. When you are able to stop needing from past people and events and to accept them for what they are, they will no longer have any power over you. When you are able to free yourself from linkages to the past, you can begin to allow a positive force to grow in your life which is based on the present, on the you who is now. New realities can be created that are based on new needs and beliefs. Now potentials can be created for the future that was not previously possible.

The past does still represent the fund of experiences that we have available to formulate our definition of self. As such, it may continue to serve as a source of enrichment for our lives without exercising a dominating influence on the present. It may even assist in the recognition of new potential for the future.

Imagine your life as being like a rope stretched out over time. Each strand of the rope could represent a different aspect of yourself, as it is expressed in your experience. The strands of the rope are interwoven with each other. At any point along the rope, some strands are visible on the surface, while other strands are buried and inaccessible. This has been illustrated in the accompanying diagram. The present could be considered as any point along the rope. At any given present moment, different aspects may be the focal point of consciousness. At one point, loneliness may be a dominant aspect, while love may rise to the surface at another time. Power may be an important aspect for a time, only to be replaced by the experience of cooperation or submission. Helplessness, pain, excitement, joy, creativity, fear, anger, hope, desperation, patience, frustration, determination, grief, and empathy are only some of the different aspects of human experience that are to be treasured.

At one time or another, for each of us, these aspects have risen to the surface and been a dominant part of our experience. The temporal gaps between the expressions of the same aspect should not disguise the interconnection of our experience through time. Our consciousness is represented by the cross-section of the rope, as possessing a wonderful capacity for a wide range of thoughts, feelings, and expression. The nature of the cross-section may change as our needs change. However, until it does, these various aspects will continue to surface at various times even though, at other times, it may seem as though they are not part of us. These hidden aspects may, in fact, be important determinants of the events that we experience.

A fuller awareness of yourself, in the present, can be gained by reawakening some of those hidden aspects through past memories. It can be an enriching and insight-provoking experience to return to some of the locations of your past, such as old homes, schools, parks, or places of employment and to try to re-experience, as vividly as possible, the memory of how you felt and thought at that time in your life. If such re-visiting is not possible, old photographs of yourself may stimulate such memories. Ask yourself whether these thoughts and feelings still contribute to your perception of reality.

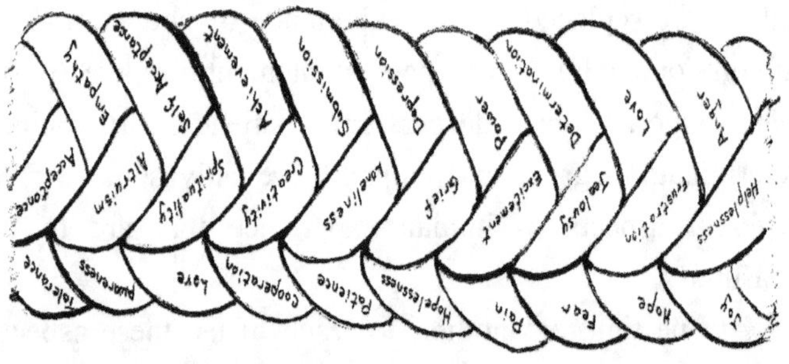

Allowing yourself to revitalize the memories of other aspects of yourself can assist you in seeing the full cross-section of your being. This is not to suggest that you should dwell upon the past. Rather, it is a suggestion that you use the richness of your past experience to reawaken the potential of aspects of yourself that you may have long forgotten. This is especially true of the more positive emotions that are often lost in adulthood. If you are able to reawaken the memory of the joy, excitement, anticipation, and wonderment that you felt at various times in childhood, you can begin to awaken that same potential for joy in the present.

This process of recall may also bring out aspects that have feelings of sadness, anger, or guilt attached to them. If so, allow yourself to experience the feelings in the context of your present needs. Look for the needs of the present that stimulate those feelings. Do not attempt to suppress those feelings; give yourself permission to experience them fully, to follow them to their most heart-rending conclusion. Let your feelings teach you about your innermost fears and about the needs and beliefs upon which these fears are based. Remember that your existence is continuous and eternal and that your needs and beliefs are only illusions of this reality.

Re-experiencing the past has two major objectives. The first is to let go of the ties that keep us from fully experiencing the present. The second is to use the past to broaden and enrich our present being. Keep these goals in mind as you make use of the exercises in this chapter.

Chapter 9
The Future

The future exists only as possibilities. It represents the totality of all of the possible events and experiences that we may create in our lives. It is the expression of the potentials that exist within us. It is infinite in its potential variety. At any point in time, we have a number of different choices available to us, each of which will take us to different destinations. We are constantly creating new futures through the choices we make.

In the previous chapter, it was suggested that you think of a child as being like a flower bed in which a variety of different seeds have been planted. Each seed represents an undeveloped potential, a capacity for experience that has not yet been discovered. This is not referring merely to the development of skills and abilities. Unfortunately, we tend to value those qualities that we feel will gain recognition and praise from those around us. In thinking about undeveloped potential, there is a tendency to seek out those attributes that could lead to fame and fortune, to become an artist, musician, athlete, intellectual, or businessman. We are, all too frequently, willing to forego our own inner assessment of our needs and to assume that, if something is valued by others, then it must be good for us.

The development of skills or abilities is a part of growth but is only a part. We start out with simple experiences that are accounted for by simple understandings. As we allow new capacities for experience to develop, our understanding expands and incorporates larger and larger parts of ourselves. As we allow ourselves to experience the many aspects of our thoughts and feelings that were described in the previous chapter, our jealousy, love, frustration, and so forth, we create the opportunity for new learning, for new understanding. When we openly receive these different aspects, we allow ourselves to see qualities that had not previously been discovered. These are the seeds of new potential for the future.

Abilities are usually thought of in terms of external reality. We value and strive to develop athletic abilities, intellectual abilities, musical abilities, and so forth. We hold in the highest regard those tangible products that can be created through the development of such skills. But abilities may also be thought of as the capacities and understandings that grow out of the exploration of new dimensions of ourselves. The capacity for empathy, the understanding and resolution of one's needs for competition, the ability to accept others as they are, the openness to express one's feelings honestly and thoughtfully, and the capability to willingly share with others are some examples of the kinds of abilities that arise out of the growth of understanding. Such abilities have a far greater impact on future possibilities than do external abilities. They shape the pattern for continuing growth so that new experiences can take place. As new inner abilities are developed, new possibilities are actually created.

For example, when the need for competition is resolved, a new future is opened up in which relationships can be experienced without comparison, in which aspects of others that have never been seen before can come forward into our perception. When this ability is achieved, a new reality is created, even though nothing in the external world has changed.

All of these abilities and potentials exist within each of us. They are the seeds of our growth. They are the vehicles by which we will each create our own future. The extent to which we develop and employ them will determine whether or not they become a permanent part of ourselves. The seeds exist but their development is not guaranteed. Seeds will grow only if they are provided with the necessary conditions to stimulate growth. Our latent understanding and the abilities that it spawns will be actualized only through our openness and willingness to strive for greater understanding. All that we are, all that we ever will be already exists. It is only the expression of those attributes that have not been fully developed.

In our experience of sequential time, we are free to choose the manner in which the expression takes place. There is no escaping from the fact that we have free will, whether we choose to exercise it or not. At the conscious level of mind, we may experience things that lead us to believe that we are the victims of circumstances. However, at a deeper level of mind, even these circumstances are of our own creation. At the conscious level of mind, we may feel we have limited choices in our actions. At a deeper level of mind, there is no limitation.

We are constantly making choices about the events we experience, even if this means that we choose to do the most habitual things. Even in sitting back and letting things happen to us, we choose the events that are most likely to occur. The limitations that we consciously experience are created through our needs and beliefs. Events that throw us up against these limitations provide the opportunity to challenge those needs and beliefs. We engage in a child's game of make-believe. Children love playing games that involve pretending that limitations exist that create problems for them to solve.

"Let's say there are alligators under the bed and we can't get off."

"Let's pretend that we have no money and we are starving."

"Let's say our parents have gone away and left us and we have to look after ourselves."

These are the games that we also engage in, through the limitations that are created by our needs and beliefs. We create the conscious illusion that some choices are not available to us, that there are certain things that we must do and some things that we must not do. We blind ourselves to the alternatives that are available. We not only insist that our needs be met, but that they should be met in the manner that we think they should be. We define a narrow path for our lives and insist that any deviation from this path will be disastrous.

How often do we stand before the future with a feeling of helplessness, feeling that we will have little to do with what happens to us? Especially in these days of burgeoning populations, it is easy to feel like an insignificant voice being swept along a river of events. There is an underlying fear that fate has already plotted our course. The power of our environment seems far greater than our capacity to direct our lives. All we can do is hope for an outcome that is favorable, trust our luck, check our astrological tables, and listen to the voices of seers and prophets. Our destiny appears to be in the hands of others.

But is it really those external circumstances that create our sense of helplessness or is it our perception of those circumstances and the limits that our perception imposes upon us? If we look at it from the other end, it is apparent that large-scale events or circumstances can affect individuals in vastly different ways. The degree to which our lives are touched by the limitations of our environment is largely determined by our recognition and acceptance of those limitations. The conduct of our daily lives is like attending a bullfight. In the center of the arena, there are some very absorbing activities taking place that are difficult to ignore. Political events, economic problems, disasters, and wars are some of the attractions of the center ring that hold our attention transfixed. All of those around us share our fascination with the color and excitement of the bullfight. The outcome seems very important to us.

However, if we begin to look around, we see that there are many other events taking place that we have ignored. We need not be immobilized by those larger events. We can begin to explore those things that are more immediately a part of our environment, learning about ourselves and those around us in a more personal way. We can begin to learn about our own inner world, about our needs and beliefs and about how we keep ourselves focused on the bullfight.

There was a time in my own life when I felt desperate about what the future would bring. Around the same time, I began to spend some time meditating each day. I used a small bronze statue as an object upon which to focus during the meditation. In time, I began to see beauty in this statue that I had never before noticed. When I was able to clear my mind of thoughts of the past and future, I allowed myself to see that statute with clarity and to see the intense beauty that existed in a simple object. Realizing this, I began to develop a greater appreciation for the beauty that exists all around us. I found it easier to accept my life as it was without needing it to be different, to look for the beauty in what is now rather than insisting that it must be different.

It is all a question of focus. If you focus on the external events, you will feel that you are limited by them, that you need them to be different in order to allow you the freedom you need. You will seek freedom externally, fantasizing about the ideal set of circumstances that would allow you to be what you want to be. This happens when you believe that there is an objective reality that is separate from your inner world; when you see a discontinuity between inner and outer. When you focus internally, on your thoughts, feelings, needs, and beliefs, you can come to see that there is no separation. Objective reality becomes an extension or projection of those inner phenomena. Limitations imposed by the environment are merely an expression of inner fears and beliefs.

Future possibilities are closed off from within. Freedom to explore future possibilities can only be created through understanding and acceptance of one's needs and beliefs. It cannot be granted by any outside force or circumstance. True freedom lies within. It is the freedom from feelings, which grows out of acceptance of self. It is the freedom from needs and from having to see the world in certain ways. It is the freedom of seeing external reality as an expression of self, of realizing that you are the creator of your own reality.

True freedom grows out of the acceptance of complete responsibility for one's own reality. If you are willing to accept full responsibility for the events of the future, you are likely to experience more of what you want more often. This does not mean that everything that happens in your life will exactly suit your tastes. There are still adversities that may be very necessary for our growth and development. In order to experience the full range of our being we must be open to all possible aspects of ourselves. Many of our capacities for experience can only be explored through events that may elicit unpleasant emotions. To be protected from such events would deprive us of the self-knowledge that comes from exploring those capacities.

We must also be willing to look at all sides of our experiences and to take as much from each experience as we can. Our conscious perception of how our needs would best be met is based on a very limited understanding of ourselves. When it seems as though life is not presenting the opportunities that we most need, we must strive for a deeper understanding of what our needs truly are. We may be focusing on needs that have little significance for our growth. We may be misunderstanding the inner needs that underlie the things that we believe we need. We may be attempting to close off areas of experience through fear and rigidity. Adversity is always experienced most acutely when there is resistance to change, when we cling to needs and beliefs, not allowing change to take place. If you can accept responsibility for the events of your life, it is possible to find opportunities for a new understanding of self in all that happens. Adversity merely opens the door to new perceptions and the exploration of new potentials. One bends like the willow in the storm when one seeks to make the best of and grow from any possible event.

Most of us are accustomed to giving responsibility for aspects of our experience to others. There are situations within which we have difficulty in seeing our own responsibility. For example, a person may be married to someone who dominates or abuses them. They may feel that they have no control over the situation and that, surely, their unhappiness is being caused by the other person. However, they do have control over the fact that their low opinion of themselves had led them to select a partner who has no consideration for their needs. Their low opinion of themselves leads to their acceptance of the abuse. It prevents them from visualizing and creating experiences in which they are respected by someone close to them. Their need for approval from others prevents them from forsaking the institution of marriage. Their fear of being unable to survive without their partner keeps them from seeking new alternatives.

If you are truly honest with yourself about the choices you have made to arrive where you are now and about the needs and beliefs that maintain the present, it will be difficult to find any situations in your life for which you are not responsible. If you are prepared to accept full responsibility for your choices, you can begin to see how you have created the reality you are experiencing. You can also see how new futures may be created through new choices. At the same time, however, keep in mind that you cannot accept responsibility for the actions of others. The actions of every individual are fully and completely his own responsibility. If you feel the need to alter the choices made by another person, you may attempt to do so. However, remember that their life is their responsibility and the final choice is theirs.

In considering future possibilities, perhaps the most important factor that limits the choices available to us is fear. Our fears tell us that there are certain possibilities that we would be incapable of coping with. The limitations that we feel are an expression of our limited awareness of different aspects of ourselves. Perhaps this could be illustrated with the following example.

Imagine Eric and Sandra, whose marriage is deeply troubled by Eric's intense feelings of suspicion and jealousy of Sandra. Underlying Eric's jealousy are strong feelings of inadequacy and worthlessness. He needs Sandra's love and support in order to retain any sense of personal worth. He fears that, without her involvement in the relationship, his life would have no value or purpose. Thus, he clings to the relationship with a desperation that is suffocating for Sandra. He needs to know her every action and requires frequent reassurance of her continued affection for him. He avoids expressing aspects of himself that she may disapprove of.

In Eric's mind, the relationship must not end because its termination would expose him to capacities or potentials within himself that he has not explored. It would bring him in touch with his loneliness and his intense need for acceptance from others. It would confront him with the fact that his unhappiness grows out of his inability to accept himself and actually has little to do with the external events of his life. As long as he is able to hold onto the relationship with Sandra, he can protect himself from these potentials. He can ignore these inner needs and pretend that his happiness depends upon Sandra's love. The idea of losing Sandra then becomes very threatening, because her loss would mean shifting from an external focus to an internal focus. It would mean taking responsibility for his experience.

Eric's fear is a reflection of the belief that certain things must not happen; that it is necessary to close off certain future possibilities. In his case, it is the belief that Sandra must not leave him. As long as his capacities for loneliness, desperation, and worthlessness remain unexplored, as long as his need for love and self-acceptance remain unresolved, he will continue to fear the possibilities that would bring him into contact with these potentials. As long as he focuses outward, toward external reality, he can avoid facing these aspects of himself. That is, provided that external reality cooperates with him.

Our fears reflect the fact that we are attempting to close off future possibilities by telling ourselves that certain things must not happen. The experience of anxiety suggests that we are not prepared to do our best to grow from and develop through anything that might happen to us. It intimates that we do not trust our ability to influence events and use our experiences to expand our understanding of ourselves.

Perhaps the ultimate fear is the fear of the termination of our own existence. Death is the thing that we strive, above all else, to avoid. Many of us avoid even thinking about it. And yet, how can life have any meaning, unless it is placed in the context of a beginning and end? By avoiding the concept of death, we leave ourselves with a limited understanding of the broad spectrum of existence. The answer to the question of what lies beyond death's door is a personal discovery. The fact that there is so little agreement may suggest that there are many equally true possibilities. It may be that what is experienced is directly determined by the beliefs of each individual. It is not my intention to attempt to put forward some ultimate explanation or theory, but merely to suggest that living life with a view to what exists beyond life is an important factor in allowing oneself to be open to experience.

Anyone who wishes to seek their own answers to this question will have no difficulty in finding a multitude of theories. Each theory carries with it its own rigidity and may place varying degrees of restriction on experience. If one is able to trust one's own inner conscience and voice, this can be used as a guide toward a concept of existence that provides an openness to life's experience. A firm conviction in one's continued existence removes the need to fear even those events that may be life threatening.

Fear or anxiety is always an indication that you are anticipating events that you are telling yourself must not happen. Instead, try exploring how these feared events might allow you to grow and develop more fully. Recognize that times of tremendous personal growth usually occur after a person allows himself (herself) to finally experience something that they have been struggling to prevent. The disaster turns out to be a new beginning. The marital separation may become the beginning of a new, fulfilling life based upon new needs. The lost job can become an opportunity to develop new skills and abilities. The feared, critical attack from another can turn into a bond of friendship based on the ability to be honest with each other.

However, such a transition can take place only when we are open to allowing it. It can only occur if we are able to let go of that which we know; if we are able to allow ourselves to experience loss. If we can let ourselves experience an uncertain future, we give ourselves more room to grow.

If a seed is planted in a forest, it will be deprived of light and will have to compete with the existing trees for space for its roots. It may grow, but it will be scrawny and weak. On the other hand, if that seed is planted after the surrounding trees have been cut down or after a forest fire has leveled the forest, it will grow to its maximum potential. So it is with our thoughts, feelings, and beliefs. There must be a breaking down of old patterns before new ones can grow. If we cling to that which is familiar, we provide no space for new possibilities.

Take some time to examine your own fears regarding the future. The following questions are ones that you may benefit from asking yourself. Writing down your answers will enhance the usefulness of the questions in stimulating your thinking about yourself.

What are some of the fears that you frequently experience? What is the worst possible outcome if each of these fears is realized?

How likely is this outcome?

How would an adjustment in your needs, values, and beliefs allow you to accept such possibilities?

What are the possible benefits of having these fears realized?

Are there future possibilities to which you feel closed, possibilities that you struggle to prevent?

What are the fears that underlie these possibilities?

Are there ways in which these feared events could be used to further your growth?

Be resolved to benefit from all your experiences. Tell yourself that you will cope with any events in a way that will enhance your development and strengthen you as a person. Remember that the future is nothing more than the myriad of possibilities that we may create through our choices. It has no power over you other than through your manner of dealing with it. Fear is merely the refusal to experience. It is a focus on the future in a negative way. There are no great pains in experience. Pain lies in anticipation.

Focusing on your needs will help you to utilize future events to maximize your growth and development. With an awareness of your needs, it is possible to extract benefits from everything that happens by looking at all sides of events. The events of your life are your own creation. But the creative process takes place on both conscious and unconscious levels. Consequently, that which you seek may arrive in the most unexpected manner. Focusing on only one future possibility places narrow limits on the means by which needs will be met.

For example, imagine Tom, who says to himself, "I need to gain self-confidence. I will feel more confident when I succeed in being promoted to a senior position at work. If I do not succeed at gaining this promotion, it will be disastrous. I must succeed in order to feel confident of my worth."

There is nothing wrong with Tom's goal or purpose, but he is placing very narrow limits on how he will gain self-confidence. He is insisting that certain events must occur in order for his needs to be met. He is likely to ignore many small opportunities to enhance his self-confidence. He might even pass up a much more effective way of filling this need because he is not looking for it. His promotion may, in fact, reduce his level of self-confidence if he has difficulty with the new job. He ignores the fact that failure to achieve his goal may result in greater self-confidence if it forces him to re-examine the value he places on other's opinions of him. He has put the fulfillment of his need in the future by suggesting to himself that nothing will happen to fill it until the anticipated event occurs.

Anytime we enter into a situation anticipating what course we want it to take or how we want it to turn out, we close ourselves off from the potential richness of the event. Only by remaining open to all possible ways of perceiving and learning from the event can we maximize our learning and development.

If, as was suggested in the chapter on the past, linear time does not exist and all events exist simultaneously, then both needs and their resolution exist at once. Whether the need is experienced or its resolution depends upon the focus of your consciousness. The resolution of needs occurs when consciousness is focused on the aspects of events that can meet the needs. As long as the focus is on the existence of needs, their continuation is guaranteed.

The suggestion that all events exist simultaneously may sound as though the future has already been determined. Perhaps in the four dimensions of space and time, which structure our reality, this is true. However, I do not believe that in the dimension of experience such predetermination exists. The meaningfulness of events, the extent to which they lead to self-awareness and self-understanding, is the variable factor. Growth does not necessarily mean an alteration of the events of your life. The growth of understanding and awareness, the changing structure of needs and beliefs, is the only real growth possible.

The events of the future are an interwoven web of possibilities that will be explored by an expanding consciousness. Choices do exist, even if the choice we make is somehow ultimately predetermined. Each person creates his own reality, with varying degrees of awareness of the creative process. The richness of experience drawn from each event will always be up to us. The extent to which we expand into the fifth dimension, that is, the quality of experience, depends upon our willingness to seek out new understandings. The nature of events is important only insofar as they lead to expanded awareness.

Chapter 10
The Present

All that ever really exists in life is the present. The past only exists through our memory. It changes as our memory changes and we seek out different confirmations about ourselves. The future only exists as possibilities that are vitalized by our needs, anticipation, and fears. The past is continually being created as lineal time flows through the present moment, just as new future possibilities are created by the choices made in the present. The present is the point of creativity.

In referring to the present, I do not mean the one or two days, hours, or even minutes that surround the present moment. The present consists of the very instant that we experience, the immediate thoughts and perceptions that are being experienced right now. Experiencing the present does not mean recalling what happened a few moments ago or anticipating what will soon happen. It consists of experiencing yourself and your surroundings as they are at this instant. It requires that you go on from moment to moment, focusing on your perceptual world as it is now.

In order to bring yourself into focus on this present moment, ask yourself what you are experiencing right now.

Look around you. What do you see, hear, smell, and feel? Try to attune your perceptions to see things as they are now, without reference to their future use or purpose and without past connotations. Be aware of yourself as you are thinking and feeling now, without thoughts about what you will be doing in the future or what you have done in the past. Seek to know yourself at this moment, as though you had no past or future.

Examine your thoughts and feelings as they are now, without reference to where they have come from or where they are taking you. At various times throughout the day, ask yourself where your attention is focused. Is it focused on the past, the future, or what is happening right now?

In general, we devote a great deal more of our attention to anything other than what is happening now. How many of us see happiness as something which always lies somewhere in the future? We tell ourselves things like:

"When I graduate, then I will be happy."

"When I get the car paid off, then I will be happy."

"When the kids are a little older, then I will be happy."

"When I get the job I want, then I will be happy."

"When I win the lottery, then I will be happy."

Happiness is seldom what we are experiencing now. Our present circumstances always seem to leave something to be desired. If only we could rid ourselves of the restrictions we feel or the burdens we carry, we would be able to really feel happy. But we see those burdens and restrictions as being imposed from outside ourselves. We attempt to separate those circumstances from our consciousness, as though we have nothing to do with their creation.

If you find yourself making statements such as the above, you can be assured that those changes in your environment will not bring the happiness you seek. Until you have learned to understand and enjoy the products of your creation, you will continue to seek something other than what you already have.

As was suggested in the two earlier chapters, all you have been and all you ever will be exists right now. Your needs exist at the same time as their resolution; pain exists at the same moment as comfort; freedom exists in concert with entrapment. What you experience depends upon your focus. When we look at a tree, we focus on the leaves rather than on the spaces between them. Why? The space between the leaves defines their shape as much as the leaves themselves. When we are injured, we focus on the pain in the injured area rather than the comfort we feel elsewhere. Does the pain dominate our consciousness or do we give it credence by concentrating upon it? When we focus on our needs, we feel the need for change in the circumstances of our lives. If we were to focus on their resolution, could we not see how they are already being met?

Life is a miraculous experience. We are surrounded by things that are so marvelous that they cannot possibly be replicated by man. Plants, animals, people, and our natural surroundings comprise a stunning world of experience. And yet we take them for granted. We want to experience the 'important' things in life, like success, fame, money, power and security. A large number of people share the belief that these are important goals, making them powerful forces in our lives. Unfortunately, these goals tend to be oriented to the future and seldom leave time for an appreciation of what is happening now. They are illusions within which we give up the creative power of our own consciousness. To hold these as goals is to place yourself at the mercy of others, and to have your worth determined by others. It is to accept the illusion that we are not free, that the reality we are experiencing is not our own creation.

Our experience in this reality is the externalization of our inner reality. It is when we lose sight of this that we are cast out of the Garden of Eden and subjected to the perils and hazards of a world over which we seem to have no control.

Thought is creative. Anything that is introduced in a physical form, into this reality is preceded by its thought form. First, the thought is conceived, and then the reality is created. All that is constant is thought. An obvious illustration of this can be found in the area of inventions. For example, the creation of the first airplane by the Wright Brothers was only accomplished because of the belief that flight was possible. At the time of their invention, this belief was coming to be widely shared. Consequently, the Wright Brothers had a fund of partially workable ideas from which they could draw to create a thought form that served as the blueprint for the final product.

It is thought that creates. When this is applied to our daily experience, we can begin to see how events and their perception are created by the beliefs we hold. Our entire reality is the enactment of our personal and shared beliefs. The greater our range of thoughts and beliefs, the wider our variety of experiences. Experiences are possible only insofar as the concept underlying those experiences exists.

All thoughts, beliefs, and needs exist only in the present. When attention is focused on the past or future, it is not possible to see the mental concepts that underlie the creative process.

It is only possible, in this way, to look at the products or potential products of creativity. Only when consciousness is fully focused on the present moment can the process of creation be known or understood. It is only now that we can know the thoughts and feelings that are creating the reality we are now experiencing.

Most of us tell ourselves that we cannot focus on the present because of the worries, troubles resentments, or problems that we have on our mind. 'How can I relax, when I know that…' I am sure that most of us could fill in that blank. Remember that in making a statement like that you are focusing your attention on a past or future event. One way to bring yourself fully into the present is to focus your attention on your body and its physical sensations. While your mind is free to explore a range of time, your body is always in the present. What is it that you are seeing? What are you touching? What are the sensations of your clothing on your body? Are there any aromas of which you are aware? Are you feeling warm or cold? How do things taste? What is the feeling of touching objects? Are there any sounds that you have been unaware of? How does your body feel? Is there tension anywhere in your body? Are you feeling pain? What parts of you feel comfortable? Are you, at this moment, actually feeling anything unpleasant? Is there actually any real discomfort now or is the discomfort you feel created by either your anticipation of the future or thoughts of the past?

It might be useful to think of your body as being like a window into this reality. It is the vehicle by which the inner self is able to interact with this reality structure. It is your tool for creative action in a reality to which it is attuned. In order to create within a physical universe, there must be an interaction between mind and body. The mind creates the thought forms and even, in many ways, creates the body. The body may impose some limitations on the conscious mind but the subconscious mind is unaffected by the body's limitations. Mind and body form an interdependent relationship to facilitate creative expression.

Take some time to notice the miraculous complexity of your body and its activity, the dexterity of your hands, your skill in balance, the amazing accuracy of your judgment in chasing a fly ball, the flexibility of your tongue in manipulating your food between your teeth, and much more. When you are able to focus on your body and its activities, sensations, and feelings, you bring yourself fully into the present.

In the present, there is seldom ever any real pain or discomfort. How many times can you recall when you would have actually experienced anything unpleasant if your attention had been fully focused on the present without reference to the future?

I think this can be illustrated by pressing a needle into your finger until the pain reaches an unbearable level. Now let someone else press the needle into your finger. I am certain that you will find that you can tolerate far more pain if you are in control of the needle. When you are in control, you know that you can stop at any time and, thus, the pain is experienced as far less severe. If another person has control of the needle, your attention is immediately thrust into the future. "What if they poke me too hard? What if they do not stop when I cannot tolerate anymore?" Such questions focus your consciousness on the anticipation of more severe circumstances in the future, making the sensations of the present more unpleasant than they need to be.

Any athlete can attest to the fact that any discomfort associated with sports is in the fear and anticipation before the event and in regrets after the event, but never in the event itself. Actions are carried out from moment to moment, in accordance with the demands of the situation, to the best of the athlete's ability. There is minimal discomfort in acting when attention is focused fully on the present. The same can be seen in emergencies, when a person may become so engrossed in the demands of the immediate moment that they lose all awareness of the past and future. Any time that one is able to become so completely oriented to the present moment, it becomes possible to experience all of the positive human emotions. Love, joy and the appreciation of the beauty that surrounds you are best experienced from the focus of the present moment.

Bringing your attention to experiences of the present will not guarantee instant nirvana or bliss. It will not result in continuous happiness at all times. However, it will facilitate changes that will bring you closer and closer to a state of self-understanding. Changes can only be made in the present. It is the only perspective through which self-acceptance can be achieved.

When you are fully aware of who you are right now, when you can truly accept yourself as you are now, without needing to be something more or less, then you can begin to experience life with a deep appreciation of all that it has to offer you.

The process of growth is itself, an illusion. By whatever process, whether through our life experiences or as an expression of our consciousness at a deeper level, we have all undergone a fragmentation of ourselves, in which we attempt to separate certain thoughts, feelings, and needs from our being.

We may, for example, refuse to acknowledge our sexual feelings, our anger toward certain persons, our fear about certain possibilities, our feelings of inadequacy, and so on. In a world of duality, we allow ourselves to become fragmented into parts of ourselves that we consider to be good and parts that we consider to be bad. We attempt to identify with those attributes that we identify as good and to dissociate from ourselves the things that we think of as bad or undesirable.

As we progress through linear time, we are confronted with the various aspects of ourselves that we are ashamed of or find difficult to accept. The thoughts associated with these fragments are the building blocks of events that we find frustrating, painful, and disappointing. These fragments stand like treacherous rocks against which the sea of life thrusts us. We break against these rocks, battered and torn until we realize that the rocks are an illusion that we have created. The pain we feel is the pain of being unable to accept our own consciousness. As our life experiences confront us with those fragments, we have the opportunity to reintegrate those unacceptable sides of ourselves and to become whole once again. Before an aspect can be integrated, it must be understood and accepted. Every new aspect that is integrated opens up new possibilities for understanding our experiences.

It expands us further into the fifth dimension, giving our experience of events a further richness.

It is interesting to consider that, regardless of whether you accept the 'Big Bang' theory of the creation of the universe as put forward by science or the notion of divine creation, creation is a process of fragmentation. Either unified matter exploded to create the universe as we know it or a unified deity fragmented His own energies to create a physical universe. Or, perhaps, both are possible. In view of this, it is interesting to consider our own fragmentation as the product of our creativity. Maybe the trials and tribulations that we wish we could avoid are, in fact, constructions of our own, which creatively elicit new potentials without ourselves. In many ways, if we could welcome the hardships and restrictions, we would be more open to seeing the new learning that those circumstances make possible. Restriction or confinement increases the need for creativity in the solution of problems. Fragmentation creates the need for reintegration and opens up a wealth of creative possibilities.

Happiness will never be a regular part of life until self-understanding is achieved. Without such awareness, there is a tendency to separate the self from events and the environment and to overlook the creative potential of the self. Self-awareness creates the possibility of recognizing the constructions of the self, of seeing reality as a personal production in which great freedom exists. When self-understanding is achieved, happiness can become an inseparable part of your experience. When all aspects of the self are understood and accepted, then there is no longer any need for fear, anger, grief, and jealousy. It is then possible for perception to expand to incorporate all events as constructions of the self through which new learning is possible.

Focusing on the present does not mean that goals are unnecessary or undesirable. Setting goals will allow you to work toward having experiences that will be helpful in expanding your understanding. Self-awareness expands your knowledge of where your potential for growth lies. For example, you may recognize feelings of anger, grief, or guilt that are, as yet, unresolved. You may have capacities for feelings that have not been developed, such as the capacity for empathy and awareness of others or the undeveloped expression of your feelings of love or of certain needs. You may have talents or abilities that could be developed or areas of experience which you have not explored.

By setting goals that involve expanding your understanding of yourself or incorporating new areas of experience, the process of defining yourself can occur more quickly and more efficiently. Because you have set goals for yourself does not mean that your attention must be focused on the future. Your goals merely direct the expression of your energies in the present. For example, if your goal is to increase your understanding of your angry feelings, then your attention will be directed toward asking yourself questions that clarify your anger rather than toward the many other ways in which you might express your anger. Such a goal allows you to bring your energies to bear on each step along the way and to fully appreciate each aspect of your experience as it leads toward the goal.

It is useful to remember that fear and anxiety are anticipatory responses and are signals that you are focusing on the future, telling yourself that certain things must or must not happen. Whenever you find yourself experiencing these emotions, ask yourself what it is that you fear. Do not give up until you have an answer. Then confront that fear. Ask yourself what is the worst possible outcome of having your fear realized. Imagine how you could cope with even that extreme possibility by understanding the beliefs behind it. How could a more flexible way of thinking about such possibilities allow you to benefit from them? Be resolved to overcome the fear.

Next, bring your attention back to what you are experiencing now. Close your eyes for a few moments and be fully aware of what you are feeling in your body. Let your focus of attention travel throughout your body and acknowledge the physical sensations that you become aware of whether they are pleasant or unpleasant. Recognize that you have created these sensations through the workings of your mind. When you recognize that you have created these physical responses, you can start to change them.

After you have begun to feel that you are in control of what is happening in your body, open your eyes and look around you. What is taking place in your immediate environment? What sights, sounds, smells, and feelings are you aware of? Take some time to fully explore and be aware of all that already exists in your perceptual world. How could you profitably expand your efforts at this moment to enhance your experience and maximize your growth and development? The only point when you can act is now. Your fears and anxieties can, in no way, change the future. It is your actions at this present moment that shape the future. The NOW is the focal point of creativity.

Consider the analogy of an artist. The information and experience gained from the past is like the paint that the artist has applied to the canvas. It can be covered but not erased. The future is the empty canvas upon which the painting will be produced. It lives only in our imagination. The present is the brush. It is that which allows the painting process to proceed. It is the focal point in which inspiration and creativity may be expressed. It is the point through which action is possible. It is the point through which action can be taken to change future possibilities. By learning to focus your attention on the present, you can begin to shape your life into what you want it to be.

Chapter 11
Dreams

In winter sleeps

The earth beneath

A blanket of fresh snow.

Full conscious still of all that will

In time, begin to grow.

And in sleep dreams of all that seems

To rise anew in spring.

In dreams, it knows

Soft winds will blow

And how the birds will sing.

In all of life

What comes through strife grows first within our dreams.

Our dreams are born when we're forlorn, dissatisfied with now.

Beneath the glove

We rise above

The way our world seems.

And find new ways

To live our days

Our dreams can show us how.

If we think of our reality as including all our experiences, we recognize that a large part of our personal reality has nothing to do with consensus reality. Much of our reality is very individual and personal. Once we move beyond our sense organs, beyond what we can see, hear, feel, taste, and smell, we enter a realm of knowledge and experience that is very unique to us. This is the realm of thoughts, fantasies, images, inspirations, intuitions, precognitions, and dreams. This is the construction zone of our waking reality.

In general, we have been taught to be suspicious and distrustful of these experiences. Our scientific society emphasizes the need for truth to be tangible, concrete, and replicable. Consequently, these other dimensions of our experience have been largely brushed aside. In doing so we have closed off important avenues of learning and creativity. It is obvious that if we are building bridges, buildings airplanes, and so on, we need to be aware of the physical laws that apply to the reality in which they are being constructed. When working in the material world, it is necessary to understand physical laws and to utilize a logic that is appropriate to those laws. However, our consciousness simultaneously spills over into many different realities. For every instance when physical laws and logic are used to limit what is possible, there exists, in our imaginations, a wealth of alternative possibilities. These imaginative alternatives also provide us with new vehicles by which to expand our experiences.

There is no need to limit or minimize the experience that we gain in the realm of dreams, fantasy, and imagination. This experience is a product of the creative function of our minds and is an expression of our mental structure, just as waking reality is. As such, it is really no different than our waking experience. The only difference is that there are certain limitations that are imposed on daily reality that do not apply to these other areas. Cause and effect logic, physical laws and temporal sequencing of events are all limitations of this reality that do not apply to other areas of mental activity. And yet, these arenas of experience are just as valid when it comes to our personal growth.

Dreams appear to have two major functions that I have been able to identify. The first is to provide experience, while the second is as a vehicle or pathway to a kind of direct learning or guidance.

The experience that is provided through dreams falls on a continuum from being very directly related to daily events to being far removed from having any direct relationship to waking reality. At this latter end of the continuum are dreams that may be highly symbolic of waking reality as well as experiences that have their own validity.

First, let us consider those dreams which are a direct reflection of daily reality. There is a certain amount of assimilation that takes place after any experience in which we mentally review the events and attempt to fit them into our existing mental structure. While our mental structure has facilitated the occurrence of certain events, those events may also have brought with them aspects that do not fit in with our existing consciousness.

Let me attempt to illustrate this with an example. Imagine Ted and Marie as a young couple who have recently married. Although they were both enthusiastic about marriage, it did not turn out as Ted had expected.

Once he is actually married, he finds it difficult to cope with Marie's need for intimacy. Ted was raised in a family in which there was very little emotional involvement between the family members. There were no outward displays of affection: problems were not openly discussed: the only feeling that was easily expressed was anger. He had hoped that marriage would meet his needs for love and acceptance. There are times when those needs are met but they are punctuated by sessions when Marie wants to know his feelings about things, when she becomes angry with him, and when she wants an intimate caring expressed in return.

Ted is frightened that his expressions of intimacy will put him in a vulnerable position. He has no experience with such behavior. His own family avoided it to such an extent that he feared something dreadful would happen if he engaged in it. He sleeps fitfully, dreaming of being smothered, of drowning, and of being chased. Marie is expressing more and more of her disappointment in his inability to provide what she is looking for in marriage. After an angry confrontation, Ted decides to leave and to bring the marriage to an end. He finds an apartment of his own and is initially relieved at not having to face Marie's demands. However, he feels despondent about the future. Subconsciously, he knows that his needs for love and acceptance cannot be met unless he is willing to face his fear of intimacy. Now when he dreams, he dreams of standing alone in the center of a large, empty stadium or of walking along a road that never ends and that leads nowhere.

Our dreams do symbolically present those aspects of ourselves that are, as yet, unresolved. Feelings that we do not yet understand and conflicts and problems, that have not yet been solved, are experienced again in our dreams, allowing us the prospect of resolving them in another reality.

Dream reality is a field for change and personal growth as much as waking reality is. Looking back to the example of Ted and his marriage nightmares, if he had been able to learn to swim in his dreams, to fight off the smothering force, or to turn and fight against that which is chasing him, he would have initiated the process of change which would have resulted in him overcoming his fears. Those dream experiences were a symbolic representation of his inner conflicts. Changing his dreams so that the conflict is overcome is just as valid as the same efforts in waking reality. His dream efforts would result in a change in his mental structure, which would lead to new experiences. Your mental structure can be affected just as significantly by dreams as by waking experiences.

I am sure that it is a rare person who has not had at least one dream in their lifetime that has had a tremendous impact on them, although they may not consciously understand its significance. I had such a dream when I was about nineteen years of age; I dreamed that I was floating on a rubber mat on a large body of water. Around me, there were other mats with people on them, some with one person on them, some with two. As we drifted along, I looked down into the water and saw a salmon swim past and made the observation that we must now be over what was the ocean. As I drifted further, the mats became more scattered and, eventually, I was alone. After a time, I drifted up to a thick cement wall that held back the water. There was a hole in the wall that looked like it had been blasted through the cement. I left my mat and crawled through the hole. On the other side was the most beautiful green grass that I had ever seen. It was about three feet high and waved in the breezes. I was awed by the beauty of this grass. Nearby, two cowboys were cutting the grass and stuffing it into a chuck wagon. They had the chuck wagon stuffed full of grass. I walked over a hill and on the other side was a scene of complete desolation. There was a village of shacks made out of rusty tin. The people of the village were cutting all the trees and burning them in long, trough-like burners. The surrounding area was denuded of trees. The ground was gray and black. What trees that were left had no branches on them and looked dead. The whole area looked like the remains of a forest fire.

I was very upset about the destruction and tried to tell the people that what they were doing was wrong. I looked across the valley and saw a wolf running among the dead trees. I told them that, if things were as they should naturally be, you should not be able to see that wolf.

I have never made any attempt to interpret that dream or to find a meaning in it. And yet I feel that the dream did have an important effect on some of the directions I took in my life. I do not mean that I had it in mind when I made choices or that its effect was a conscious one. However, I believe that the dream was an expression of what my purpose in life was and who I wanted to become. The dream served as a crystallization of my purposes, although I had a very long way to go to achieve those ends. However, at that time, I had no conscious awareness of any of the things which I am saying now. I did not have to have a conscious understanding for the dream to do its work. The dream subconsciously catalyzed my desire to avoid destructive ways of life and opened my eyes to the richness that could exist if I were to do that. The dream initiated a process of change which was to take place over a period of years.

The experiences that are presented in dreams such as this certainly have value in their own right without needing to be translated into the language of cause and effect. Conscious recall of such dreams adds to the richness of the experience and allows for further utilization of the events of the dream to create changes in one's mental structure. The events of dreams can add tremendous variety to our range of experiences because they do go beyond the limitations that we experience in our daily lives. I would like to illustrate this with some more examples taken from my personal dream records.

1 January 1980: I have only a dim memory of the place that I was in. I know that what was important in this place were thoughts. While I was there, I met someone who was looking for a gift for another. There was a pond there, such as you might find in the lobby of a large office building or hotel. This person was looking in the pond for something to give. I tried to show them a beautiful little gift that functioned as a clock. It consisted of several small cubes which you threw into the water. The fish would move them in such a way as to tell the time. However, this person seemed lost and confused and could not understand the nature of the gift. He had been looking for something bigger and flashier. He left disappointed.

Another person passed by who wandered along like a zombie. I tried to communicate with him but he was not interested in listening. He went to wait for an elevator and I was concerned that he might commit suicide by jumping from an upper story. A friend appeared and said that he would help look after the person. The dream ended with me holding in my hands a beautiful golden box. I knew that contained within the box was a thought. It was a much-cherished possession.

This dream reinforced in my mind, in a very powerful way, the idea that thoughts are the most valuable possession that we have. We use them to construct our reality. The process of personal growth is totally guided by our thoughts. The expression of these ideas was more effective in this brief dream than it could ever have been in waking reality.

The next dream is one that I feel illustrates the flexibility and freedom that we have in dreams to manipulate and change our experiences and try out different solutions to problems. We may even present challenges to ourselves to work on in dreams.

10 November 1980: I dream that I am standing on a hill overlooking a valley. There is an earthquake. The earth is shaking violently. Across the valley is a large dam among the mountains and I can see the water splashing above it. Some of the water is spilling over the dam and I think of the possibility of the dam bursting. I am concerned about the welfare of Terry (my wife) and our children who are in a nearby city. I walk back to the city after the shaking stops. On my arrival there, I think about how nearly impossible it will be to find them. Buildings have fallen down. I don't even know where to look. As I walk along the street looking for them, I notice a crowd of people ahead.

Terry and the children are in the crowd. I am very happy to see them. At this point, I became aware of having the dream and thought about how easy it was to get from where I was to the city. I wondered what it would be like if it hadn't been so easy. I wanted to make it more challenging. I begin dreaming again and find myself back on the hill, but this time the easy path back to the city is blocked off by landslides. I have to go the opposite way which involves crawling across some rooftops that drop onto a balcony that has windows into a warehouse. In the warehouse is an elevator that will take me down but first I have to find a way into the warehouse. The dream ended here because of the need to get up.

Remember, dream reality and waking reality are both expressions of your mental structure. As such, they are both valid arenas for experience. The problem-solving that you do in your dreams is no less valid than that which you do in daily life. The experiences that you have in dreams can contribute to your growth as much as daily experience. The only difference between waking and dreaming realities is the limitations that are applied to them. In waking reality, we experience the expression of our mental structure as though it were not a part of us, as though we were separated from those expressions of ourselves. We apply limitations to our experiences that enhance the feeling of separation between ourselves and our reality. We apply limitations of cause and effect logic, temporal sequencing, and physical laws to a greater extent than we need to.

In dreams, we are free to drop these limitations and to express our consciousness in a free-flowing form that is more in tune with the true nature of the inner self. The inner self consists of energy that knows no limitations. It freely creates a reality where thought and form are one and the same. This reality is available to us in our dreams and can be used for our growth.

The second function of dreams, which was mentioned earlier, is as a vehicle for a kind of direct guidance or instruction. I do not pretend to know how this takes place but I have had a number of such dreams that have convinced me that direct learning can take place through dreams. I will share a number of examples to provide a better idea of what I am talking about.

3 January 1980: This dream is difficult to really describe other than to say that it left me with a strong feeling that I can make things happen in my life. It was just some square buttons of light that went off and on. They also had depth to them.

8 January 1980: The dream was something to the effect that people are like slot cars, driving along in their slots with their destiny totally determined. This was more in the sense that they let their lives be totally guided and determined by the forces of society and the world around them. There is no creativity in the way they live.

15 January 1980: I woke out of a deep sleep to the sound of the alarm. I could only remember that in the dream a voice was saying that just because life is an illusion; it does not mean that you should not take it seriously. Life is a special opportunity for learning and experience.

25 January 1980: I woke up at 4:30 with no real recollection of what I had been dreaming, but having a thought clearly in mind. The thought was that each person holds full responsibility for the choices in their life and that this is something that should not be interfered with.

2 February 1980: I awoke with the thought in my mind about developing new pathways in my brain. After thinking about it for a few minutes, I began to think of the brain as a microcosm of universal knowledge. Each thought opens a new pathway within the brain. If all the brain pathways were developed, total understanding would be obtained.

3 February 1980: I dreamed of what was like a large disc that created a force field. There appeared to be six parts to this force field. It was as though this force field was being applied to our world by a greater spiritual force.

3 March 1980: In the dream, there were flashing lights blinking on and off. They were part of a panel. At the same time, a voice was saying, "Now you can begin to use your full potential." I awoke. It was 4:30 a.m. As I lay in bed, this thought kept running through my mind.

September 1980: I had been somewhat concerned about violence, especially after watching the Shogun series on television. As I awoke one morning, a voice was saying, "Some people need to experience violence in order to learn."

29 November 1980: I dreamed of going through a kind of warp wherein I moved from one reality to another. It was a strange experience that was somewhat like going through the wringer of a washing machine.

7 December 1980: I dreamed of how events are formed or created in this reality. It was clear at that time but could not be brought back into the terms of our reality easily. It was something like putting on a coat.

Dreams such as these have always shared a number of characteristic qualities. Whenever I have such a dream, I have no clear perception of any surrounding environment in the dream. Whereas other dreams take place against a background of mountains, buildings, and so forth, these dreams have no distinguishable features in the background. The content frequently seems clear in the dream but is difficult to translate into terms of our reality. There is more uncertainty as to the actual events of the dream. Such dreams are frequently accompanied by a voice that makes statements that are usually relevant to my personal growth.

In order to theorize about the nature of such dreams, I must emphasize that I see man as a multidimensional being, existing on many different levels of consciousness simultaneously. There is a part of our consciousness that exists on the level of our daily interaction in the reality we focus on. There is also a part of us that communicates with plants, animals, and minerals, even though we are not conscious of this communication. Further, there is a part of us that stretches beyond this material reality into other realms of experience.

Although we exist at all levels, our consciousness determines the focal point of our involvement at any point in time. When we dream, we focus our consciousness on those other realms. I emphasize the plural here since I do believe that there are several distinct levels of consciousness, each emphasizing different aspects of reality. In each realm, we communicate with the minds of others who share that reality. Thus, I believe that dreams such as the ones I have described do represent an interchange of information with the minds of others who have a different kind of awareness than I do.

I once brought this subject up with Zasep Tulku Rinpoche, a Tibetan Buddhist monk, who lived in a nearby town. He indicated that the Tibetan Buddhists recognize three types of gurus or teachers. Those are:

1) Internal guru through your own wisdom you act as your own guru. This is possible when you have become awakened.
2) External guru, a spiritual teacher in this reality.
3) Spirit guru, a spirit acts as the guru, especially through dreams.

I found this information to be an interesting supplement to my own thoughts on the matter.

The major barrier that most of us have in utilizing dreams to expand our personal growth is our reluctance to treat them with any degree of importance. I can certainly speak from experience, as for several years, I treated dreams as being curious artifacts of our nervous system that did not warrant the time and trouble to even try to remember. For a long time, my only response about dreams was that I did not have any. When I learned that everyone dreamed for several hours each night, my response changed to announce that I never remembered my dreams.

I scoffed at the idea of studying dreams in my psychology courses because I could not remember my dreams, and, when I did, they were so confusing, that attempting to understand them made me feel quite inadequate. I did not like things that I felt I could not understand. But I was safe because most of my professors seemed to feel that way too. As I have learned to be more flexible in dealing with my experience, it has become easier to incorporate the experience of dreams into the creation of my conscious reality.

One of the annoying aspects of dreams is that, in dreams, we always seem to be confronted with aspects of ourselves that we would rather not acknowledge. We find ourselves face-to-face with our fears or with feelings that we do not understand and are trying to ignore. In dream reality, all aspects of ourselves are striving to be incorporated through understanding and acceptance. In dream reality, we are striving to be complete beings with no unresolved feelings or unfulfilled needs. This is also true for waking reality. However, in our daily lives, it is easier to separate ourselves from our creation and to ignore aspects of ourselves. Thus, the conscious utilization of dreams to enhance personal understanding can be an excellent avenue for personal growth. In order to use dreams in this way you must be willing to acknowledge the events of dreams as an expression of aspects of your consciousness and to work toward resolution of those dream events with as much vigor as you would use in your daily life. Remember, they have equal validity.

The exercises that follow are designed to assist you in making greater use of your dream reality. They presume a starting point that is similar to my own. That is, they are designed to assist someone who is beginning with the habit of totally ignoring their dreams so that they have no conscious memory of them. If this is not your starting point, then you may wish to begin further along in the series of exercises.

Exercise 1: Achieving conscious recall of dreams

The failure to recall dreams is a habit just like the habit of forgetting people's names after you are introduced to them. Changing the habit begins with telling yourself that it is important that you remember. Before you go to sleep at night, tell yourself that you will make a determined effort to remember your dreams. When you wake in the morning, do not immediately orient yourself to your surroundings. There is a balance point in your consciousness where you can go either way. You can go back into your dreams or you can bring yourself fully out of sleep and into daily reality. Try to find that balance point.

When you have found it, let yourself remain at that point while you ask yourself what you were dreaming. Do not bring yourself fully out of sleep before you do this or the dreams will be lost. As soon as you involve yourself in thoughts about the day ahead, it will be difficult to retrieve dream memories. From the balance point, let yourself recall as many dreams as possible. Review the dreams from beginning to end and be sure that you recall them completely. Then bring yourself out of sleep and you will retain the memory clearly. Going back to sleep at this time will jeopardize the memory. If you must go back to sleep, take a few moments to write the dream down.

If you keep a pencil and paper next to your bed, it will be easy to jot down a description of the dream. Do not be discouraged by initial failures. Your ability to remember your dreams will grow with continued effort.

Exercise 2: Keeping a dream diary

A dream diary can be a helpful tool in expanding your awareness and understanding of your dreams. Recording some of your dreams allows you an opportunity to think more intently about their significance. Symbolism is a natural quality of dreams and a dream record can be helpful in interpreting some of the symbols. You may notice certain symbols being repeated and this might draw your attention to how symbols are used in your own dreams. Although I recommend the recording of some dreams, I do not feel that it is desirable to attempt to keep a comprehensive dream diary. There must be a balance between the amount of time spent doing something and its benefit.

To painstakingly record every dream is no more desirable than to write down everything that happens in your daily life. If you allow yourself to be lazy about recording you will find that there are some dreams which are really worth recording and many that are not. Those less significant dreams can be orally shared with an interested friend or spouse and can serve as food for thought during the following day, whereas dreams that were very striking should be recorded. This is especially true for dreams of guidance.

Exercise 3: Expanding conscious participation in dreams

It is possible to consciously participate in and change the events of dreams. Even when a dream has been completed, it can be repeated with changes and alterations being made to it. In order to do this, you must expand your capacity to consciously participate in your dreams.

This is known as lucid dreaming, a skill that requires some determined effort to achieve. If you have used the first two exercises to become more aware of your dream, you will find that there are times when your consciousness is very close to the dream. You may feel, as you sit on your balance point, that you could go back into a dream and be consciously involved in it. As you are mentally reviewing the dream, it may become vivid enough that you feel that you are re-experiencing it. However, this time you are able to ask yourself, "What would have happened if I had done this or that?" As you ask such questions, the possibilities may begin to unfold.

You may also find that there are times when you come close to waking consciousness during a dream and gain the awareness that you are participating in a dream. From this state, you can begin to will certain events in the dream. Either of these possibilities will occur more frequently if you will them to. If you tell yourself before going to sleep that you will strive for conscious awareness of your dreams, you will achieve this state more readily.

Exercise 4: Manipulating dream events

With sufficient expansion of your awareness of participation in dreams, you can begin to alter the events of your dreams. This is an important step which can greatly facilitate your personal growth. Keep in mind that dreams represent your attempts to resolve and integrate conflicting needs and feelings. For example, being chased by something dangerous in your dreams likely represents your fear of some need or feeling. You run from it in your dreams and you do not know how to cope with it in your daily life. How you attribute cause and effect depends upon where you place the emphasis. If, in your dreams, you can change the events so that the problem is removed or resolved, you will have mentally begun to accept and integrate the feelings that are symbolized in the dream conflict.

As you experiment with your ability to manipulate dream events, you are likely to find that you may do this either by allowing the dream to run to completion and then exploring alternatives or by consciously shaping the course of the dream as you progress through it. This latter ability may take some time to develop.

If you can accept that your existence transcends birth and death, it becomes easy to see that your life in this reality is really a dream. Dreams have a beginning and an end, as does our experience here. Each of our lives is an expression of an entity whose existence extends beyond this reality. That entity, which is the inner self, knows no beginning or end. The events of our lives are symbolic expressions of the inner self as it interacts with the material world through the mental structure it has formed, just as dreams are its symbolic expression in a reality where thought and form are the same. Life in this reality is a dream in which the inner self is symbolically expressing itself. Growth in this reality contributes to the growth of the inner self. Growth of the inner self creates changes in this reality.